Medical English Test System(METS)

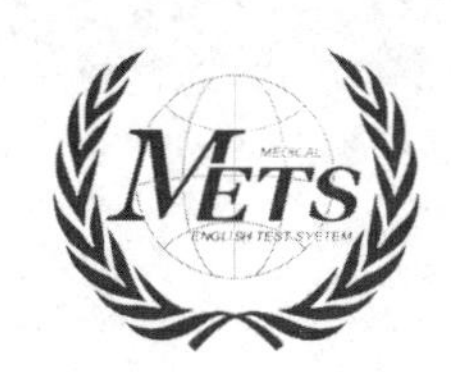

医护英语水平考试办公室
医护英语水平考试教研中心 组织编写

METS
测试与评析
（二级）
Level 2

主　编　刘新民　高　丽
（以下排名以姓氏笔画为序）
副主编　任莉枫　张　莹　张　捷
　　　　赵　旦
编　者　王宗忠　李　静　陈冶彬
　　　　陈　烨　张　倩　沈　艳
　　　　周思源　罗　渝　殷　丹

南京大学出版社

图书在版编目(CIP)数据

METS测试与评析. 二级 / 刘新民，高丽主编. -- 南京：南京大学出版社，2018.6(2024.3重印)
ISBN 978-7-305-20089-2

Ⅰ. ①M… Ⅱ. ①刘… ②高… Ⅲ. ①医学—英语—水平考试—自学参考资料 Ⅳ. ①R

中国版本图书馆CIP数据核字(2018)第069685号

出版发行 南京大学出版社
社　　址 南京市汉口路22号　　　　邮　编 210093

书　　名 METS测试与评析(二级)
METS CESHI YU PINGXI(ER JI)
主　　编 刘新民　高　丽
责任编辑 刁晓静　　　　　　编辑热线 025-83592123

照　　排 南京南琳图文制作有限公司
印　　刷 南京百花彩色印刷广告制作有限责任公司
开　　本 787×1092　1/16　印张 9.75　字数 224 千
版　　次 2018年6月第1版　2024年3月第2次印刷
ISBN 978-7-305-20089-2
定　　价 35.00元

网址：http://www.njupco.com
官方微博：http://weibo.com/njupco
微信服务号：njuyuexue
销售咨询热线：(025) 83594756

前言

《METS测试与评析》1—4级系列丛书由医护英语水平考试办公室和医护英语水平考试教研中心组织编写，全国近20所各类医学院校50余名教师和专家参加编写和审稿工作。丛书对各级别METS考试的特点分别进行综述，其中的相关试题严格按照2017年最新版《医护英语水平考试考试大纲》的要求进行设计，辅以较为详尽的分析和说明，并提供参考答案和作文范文，旨在帮助学生有效备考，顺利通过医护英语水平考试各级别的考试。本系列丛书既可供学生自主学习使用，又可以用作METS考试强化教材，也是英语教师开展METS考试研究的重要参考资料。

参加编写《METS测试与评析》(二级)的教师包括：主编：刘新民(南京医科大学康达学院)、高丽(南京医科大学)；副主编：任莉枫(钟山职业技术学院)、张莹(四川省雅安职业技术学院)、张捷(上海健康医学院)、赵旦(无锡卫生高等职业学校)；编者：王宗忠(上海健康医学院)、李静(河南省漯河医学高等专科学校)、陈冶彬(无锡卫生高等职业学校)、陈烨(无锡卫生高等职业学校)、张倩(上海健康医学院)、沈燕(钟山职业技术学院)、周思源(南京医科大学)、罗渝(广州医科大学)、殷丹(常州卫生高等职业技术学校)。

目　录

METS 二级考试综述

根据2016版医护英语水平考试(METS)新大纲,METS 二级考试(笔试)由听力(Listening)、阅读与写作(Reading and Writing)两部分构成。考试时间为120分钟,满分为100分。试卷结构,包括题型、题量、赋分、权重、考试时间等如下表所示:

	测试任务类型		为考生提供的信息	题目数量	原始分数	权重(%)	考试时间(分钟)
Ⅰ. 听力	Part One	信息匹配	短对话	5	5	30	20
	Part Two	信息判断	长对话	5	5		
	Part Three	多项选择	长对话	5	5		
	Part Four	填写表格	长对话	5	5		
Ⅱ. 阅读与写作	Part One	信息匹配	段落	10	10	50	70
	Part Two	信息判断	短文	10	10		
	Part Three	多项选择	短文	5	5		
	Part Four	补全短文	短文	5	5		
	Part Five	填词补文	短文	10	10		
	Part Six	短文写作	表格等	1	15	20	30
总计				60+1	75	100	120

为了帮助考生复习应考,我们将试卷的两部分简述如下,内容包括考试要求、题型分析、真题简评、应试技巧介绍等。

一、听力(Listening)

根据新大纲要求,听力测试由4部分组成,每部分5题,共20题,主要考查考生理解口头信息的能力。本部分考试时间为20分钟,分数权重为30%。

Part One 信息匹配

第一部分为5段医患或护患之间的简单对话(共约200词),要求考生根据听到的信息辨识对话中"病痛"或"问题"这类特定信息,并将这种信息与5位患者的名字相匹配。在给出的8个选项中,1个为示例答案,另有2个为干扰项。每段对话之间有3秒钟的间隔供考生答题。录音播放两遍。

从近几年的全真题来看,开篇的5段对话均较容易,内容则为医生或护士询问病人病情或需要解决的问题,由一男一女读2～3个来回;而有关疾病、症状或疼痛部位等的医学词汇亦较为常见,如 fever, cough, dizzy, influenza, stomachache, nausea, insomnia, diarrhea, loss of appetite, in the knee, in the throat, around the hip 等。因此,考生只要掌握基本的医学词汇即能解题。具体说来,考生要充分利用播放指示语的时间迅速扫视8种病痛名称,若有患者名字,则亦应尽快记住这些名字;其次,要正确进行患者与病痛之间的匹配,关键是要听懂患者讲述自己病痛的关键语句,方能对号入座。其实,在本题的5组对话中,患者均明确说出自己的病痛,无需考生推测,故利于考生作答。

Part Two 信息判断

本部分要求考生根据听到的一段医患或护患之间的长对话(约250词),对相关事实性信息作出正误(True or False)判断。这段录音播放两遍,每遍播完后有5秒钟的间隔供考生答题。

信息判断题由于对话较长,难度自然有所加大;历年真题亦反映了这一特点。与 Part One 相比,除了语言稍难,内容也更复杂。以往真题内容曾涉及 breast cancer, prescription filling, insomnia, headache, admission, observation 等。考题设计则多为对事实或细节的正误判断,如:"The liquid drug should be shaken well before use." "The nurse wants to have a talk with James' wife." "After taking sleeping pills, she was able to sleep well."等;鲜有推理题或篇章题。可见,考题设计的难度并不大;考生若能把握对话的细节,或对某个问题的事实性陈述,解题便不困难。

Part Three 多项选择

本部分要求考生根据听到的一段医患或护患之间的长对话(约300词),辨识重要或特定的细节内容,并从所提供的3个选项中选择一个最佳答案。录音播放两遍,每遍播完有5秒钟的间隔供考生答题。

Part Three 其实是由 Part Two 演变而来,二者既有相似之处,亦有诸多不同。相似之处在于,二者的文本均为长对话,且考题均以事实题、细节题为主;而不同之处则在于 Part Two 文本长度约为250词,而 Part Three 则约为300词;Part Two 为正误判断题(True or False),而 Part Three 则为多项选择题。显然,Part Three 要难于 Part Two。反观近年真题,命题思路与前述基本吻合,而文本内容则多为疾病检查、疾病症状、病人护理、治疗措施等。如前所述,Part Three 的考题多为事实题、细节题,如:"Where does the patient feel the pain?" "What kinds of exams has Mr. Jones received recently?" "Which body system do Robert and his doctor talk about?"等。对于这类多项选择题考生并不陌生,因阅读测试亦有此类试题。解题关键仍是听懂有关考题的关键信息,尤其是疾病名称、症状、疼痛部位、治疗措施、时间地点等。

Part Four 填写表格

本部分要求考生根据听到的一段医患或护患之间的长对话(约300词),辨识重要或特定的信息，并根据听到的信息填写表格。这段录音播放两遍，每遍播完有5秒的停顿时间供考生答题。

从近几年的真题来看，这部分均为病人登记表，内容包括患者姓名、年龄、职业、主诉、治疗措施及注意事项等，要求考生根据所听到的信息填写表格中删去的5个词或短语。一般而言，这些删去的词或短语多数较为简单，如：heart，July 10，pressure，positive等，但有些则不易拼出，如：allergic，tablets，ulcer等，可谓难易结合，以易为主。与听力的前三部分相比，第四部分不仅要求考生听懂相关信息，而且要求考生能拼出所需填写的词语；而拼写无疑是考生的弱项，这是第四部分的难点所在。在实考时，考生应在播放指示语时迅速浏览考题，以便对表格中的文字有一个基本的了解，从而预估考题内容，填出相关词语，这是解题的关键所在。

学习建议：

二级听力试题共四个部分：信息匹配、信息判断、多项选择和填写表格。我们在前面对上述各部分的题型及解题技巧等作了简略说明。这里尚有几点要再次强调一下。首先，要充分利用发考卷后，放考题提示的一段时间，快速阅读Part One的5题题干，尽量记住5个病人的病痛，为答题作好准备；同时，本部分若有病人的名字，亦须记住，以便与各自病痛匹配。看完Part One的5题后，如果时间仍有富余，自应再读Part Two的5题信息判断题，争取对前两部分的10题有一个初步的印象，从而预测录音内容，提高答题准确率。Part Three是多项选择题，在放指示语时，考生不仅应迅速阅读本部分5个句子，亦应浏览每题中的3个选项，并作出合理预测。Part Four是填写表格，解题关键在于拼写词语，考生应在平时重视单词的读音和拼写，方能正确填写词语。

其次，在听录音时，最好能适当记录；用符号或字母记下相关的数字、人名、地名、关键词、重要的细节等，以便答题时有据可依。

第三，答题时要当机立断，相信第一感觉，切忌犹豫不决，反反复复，贻误全局。

上述听力技巧自然有助于我们提高解题的正确率，但是，若无平时持之以恒的听力训练，任何技巧都于事无补，不能奏效。因此，为了提高听力，考生平时应多看、多听英语节目，如CGTN(China Global Television Network)、CRI (China Radio International)、VOA、BBC等。只要持之以恒，坚持半年、一年，听力必有长进。

二、阅读与写作(Reading and Writing)

阅读与写作测试由6个部分组成，前5部分为阅读测试，第6部分为写作测试。阅读的5个部分主要考查考生理解书面信息的能力。这部分考试时间为70分钟，分数权重为50%。

Part One　信息匹配

本部分考查考生对一篇医学短文(约350词)略读与寻读的能力。近几年的全真题均为6段文字，内容涉及专题阐述，如estrogen(雌激素)，first aid等，或是6个病例关于疾病或症状等的描述，如six symptoms of hormone imbalance，six kinds of coughs，health hazards in daily life，various cancer symptoms等。6段文字后有10个问题或陈述，这些问题或陈述均涉及 6 段文字中的某些细节,如:"Which part mentions that eating at your office can increase your strss level?" "Point out which case mentions the one who suffered from tiredness with no obvious cause." "Which kind of coughs ends with a rattle or wheeze?"等。要求考生将 10 个问题或陈述与 6 段文字的某一细节,如疾病、症状、疼痛部位等进行匹配。由于段落数少于问题数,故某个段落可与一个以上的问题或陈述配对。

这类题目主要考查考生对文章细节的把握;因此,解答这类题目可按照定位→扫读→答题的顺序,先评估并选定每一题中的关键词或信号词(这与个人的认知和判断力紧密相关),再用扫读的方法快速浏览包含该关键词或信号词的段落,一旦找到,迅速答题。至于题目的顺序是否与段落的顺序相同则因题而异,若二者相同,则解题要容易得多;但在很多情况下,二者的顺序并不一致,增加了解题的难度。

Part Two 信息判断

本部分考查考生理解常见医学短文(约 350 词)中明确或含蓄表达的重要信息的能力。题目要求考生在读懂全文的基础上,对给出的 10 个句子作出正确(True)、错误(False)或未提及(Not Given)的判断。

近年来的全真试卷中,这部分的内容较为广泛,如有关 Ebola, high blood pressure, silicone breast implants 等,还有关于医疗文化方面的短文,如 disadvantages of high heels, the development of nursing 等。从考题来看,真题中仍以细节题居多,如:"Less than 286,000 women had cosmetic surgeries in the U. S. during 2014." "It is advised that you should keep heels no more than 4 cm." "The immune response that the vaccine generates has been measured for more than a year."等。

正误判断题与匹配题一样,亦是在传统的多项选择题基础上发展而来,目前已成为诸多考试的主流题型之一。这种题型除 True, False (或 Right, Wrong) 以外,尚有 Not Given(或 Not Mentioned, Doesn't Say 等)这一选项。就解题技巧而言,判断一个句子"对"或"正确",这与做一般的多项选择题类似;但判断一个句子是"错",还是"未提及"则比较困难。一般说来,所谓"错",一定是针对文中某个正确的陈述的错误,与这个正确的陈述唱反调,即所谓"一正一反",二者仍然紧密相关;而"未提及"则与文章没有任何正面或反面的联系,即所谓"风马牛不相及"。当然,在有些情况下,判断"错"与"未提及"是比较困难的。二者可能会互相误判,即"错"的可能会误判为"未提及",反之亦然。这就要求我们加强训练,提高对二者区别的敏感度。

Part Three 多项选择

本部分考查考生理解常见医学短文(约 350 词)中明确或含蓄表达的重要信息的能力,以及归纳主旨大意的能力。题目要求考生在读懂全文的基础上,从每题所给的 3 个选项中选出最佳答案。

多项选择题是一种容量大、考察面广的题型,其考查内容包括篇章、词汇、语法等方方面面,因而是各级各类英语考试的一个传统题型,也是一个重要题型。METS 考试也采用了这种题型。近年来 METS 这部分真题内容广泛,有医学专题文章,如 cardiac arrest, plasma therapy 等,亦有医疗科普文章,如有关 losing weight, benefits of being scared 等,甚至还选取了一些医学故事，如“Yoga Saved My Life”等。这部分的考题设计亦较为多样，有细节题，如：“The heart muscle receives oxygenated blood from ________.”“Which of the following is not mentioned as the doctor's advice of a safe weight loss?”；亦有篇章题，如：“Which of the following statements is true according to the passage?”“What is the author's attitude towards the haunting experiences?”；间或还可见词汇题，如：“What does the underlined word decline mean in the last paragraph?”等。由此可见，多项选择题较为灵活、实用，亦较为复杂。要做好这一题型，考生应具有较为扎实的英语语法知识和相当数量的词汇，还应具有较强的对语言意义的领悟、判断与运用的能力。当然，在应试情景下，解答多项选择题最直接、最简单的方法就是迅速锁定题干所表达的含义；即根据具体情况，将题干的意思与文章中的某一个词、某一个句子，或某一段话对接，然后运用直接选择法、排除法、比较法或逻辑推理法确定正确答案。

Part Four　补全短文

本部分考查考生理解常见医学短文(约 200 词)篇章结构的能力。这类文章通常介绍某种医学操作流程，文中留有 5 处空白，文章后给出 6 个句子，要求考生根据每处空白的上下文或通篇含义，选择一句合适的句子填入该空白。所选文章结构严谨，层次分明，逻辑性强，能较好地检测应试者把握文章总体结构及上下文逻辑关系的能力。

近几年的真题内容涉及 how to use a peak flow meter, how to deal with nosebleeds, how to take a blood sample, how to wash hair in bed 等。这种有关程序的文章多为祈使句组成，如：“Roll up your sleeves.”“Take a deep breath.”等；而应填入的句子有的在一个程序的最后，如：“Stand up straight. (47)...”有的在某一程序的开头，如：“(49)... Write down the number where the indicator tab stopped.”有些在中间，如：“Inhale medication. Upon full exhalation, place the DPI mouthpiece into your mouth with a good seal between your lips. (49) ... Count to 10 slowly while holding your breath.”还有些则为整个程序，如：“(50)...”等。应该说，补全短文题是较难的一种题型。要正确解答这一题型，考生首先应加强对语篇的理解，尤其是对文章的脉络和逻辑关系的把握。其次，在正确理解上下文的基础上，考生应有较强的预测能力，善于估猜空白处可能的句意，然后快速阅读给出的 6 个句子，选定最合适的一句。

Part Five　填词补文

本部分通过词汇考查考生理解篇章的能力。题目要求考生通读一篇约 300 词的短文(被删掉 10 个词)，然后根据上下文从所给的 12 个单词中选择一个正确的词填入相应空白处，其中有 2 个为干扰项。

所谓填词补文，即完形填空题。这种题型早已成为各级各类英语考试的重要题型。它强调考生对整体语篇的把握，着重考查考生综合运用语言知识的能力，包括语法结构分析能力，词语辨析能力，语篇理解能力，逻辑推理能力等；是一种有一定难度的障碍性阅读理解题。METS 近几年的真题均为医学短文，如 drug dosage, hand washing, medical teams, the circulatory system, the hidden danger of chronic pain 等，语言难度适中。所考词汇有名词、代词、动词、形容词、副词、连词、介词、分词等，可谓词类全覆盖。12 个单词难易搭配，但多为较容易的词,如:way, try, care, team, sense, repeat, raise, generally, role, disease, capacity, limit 等;当然也有少数稍难些的词,如 component, professional, fatal, optical, calculate, shrug, infectious, diagnosis 等,但所占比例较小,约十之二三。

怎样做完型填空?一般有两个基本方法,一是先通读全文,弄清文章的大概意思,然后根据文章的主旨和发展脉络,逐一答题。另一种方法是不看全文,仅看首句和第一、二空便开始逐一答题。两种方法各有利弊,主要看个人习惯。无论采用哪种方法,重要的是理解全文,尤其是根据空白处的上下文预测该空白应填词语的词性和语法形式,以缩小选择范围。这是做完型填空的重要技巧之一。此外,答题时还要注意文章与题目、题目与题目间的照应关系,要前后参照,上下贯通,选择符合上下文的选项。

Part Six 写作

本部分考查考生书面表达的能力,要求考生根据试题所提供的信息撰写一篇约 100 词的短文。这部分考试时间为 30 分钟,分数权重为 20%。

近年来的写作真题均为表格题,即由英文单词、短语和检测数据等构成的病人入院报告、出院小结、诊疗方案等。这类表格题通常提供较为详细的患者信息,包括姓名、性别、年龄、入(出)院日期、病情、医学检查、诊断、治疗及注意事项等,考生只要将所给词语扩展成句,便可成文。因此,做这种表格题要比命题作文容易。值得注意的是,考生应该按照表格各项内容的顺序,将主要信息扩词成句,最后成文。一般而言,若字数允许,应将表格中所给信息全部写入文章。当然,若所给信息较多,考生则应有所选择,以免包罗万象,徒增错误,或超过字数过多。这里尤应强调,考生要有扎实的英语功底,因为这是应对任何考试,任何考题的不二法宝。

学习建议:

1. 阅读

METS 的阅读理解与其他英语考试一样,占比最大。以二级为例,其阅读部分共 5 项任务:信息匹配、信息判断、多项选择、补全短文和填词补文;题量多,分值高,权重大,是整个考试的重中之重。只有做好阅读,方能顺利过关。如何做阅读题?有人认为,应先通读全文,明确结构,把握主题,了解细节,然后做题;但这种方法耗时较多。还有人认为,应先看题,带着问题再读文章。这种方法较为省时,但可能只适合那种考题和文章内容顺序完全一致的情况,如果题目顺序和文章内容的顺序不一致,这一方法恐难奏效。再说,有些问题,诸如中心思想题、推论题等必须读完全文才能答出。以上两种方法各有利弊。考生可否采用第三种方法,即"边读边做"的方法。具体说来,考生读完第一段或者三五行就看第一题,或其他题目,看哪一题能和已读过的内容挂上钩(当然要排除中心思想、作者态度等一类有关全文的题目),若不能匹配,则继续往下读。这样或许可以明确目标,节约时间。

当然,做好阅读最为重要的仍然是基本功。考生应大量记忆词汇和短语,努力扫除阅读中的词汇障碍。同时,还要认真学习语法,包括时态、语态和句子的结构,提高分析句子结构的能力,从而提高阅读理解能力。

2. 写作

写作是检测考生语法、词汇、逻辑思维等综合能力的一种产出性活动。其重要性越来越受到人们的重视。METS 四个级别均设有写作测试,考生应加强写作练习,提高写作能力。关于写作技巧和写作中应注意的问题，前面已有评述，下面再补充几点，供考生参考。

(1) 关于分段

二级写作要求考生写100词。若考生仅写一段，也无可厚非。如写两段，或两段以上，就要注意分段。英语中有两种规范的分段法：一种是空格不空行，即每段开头空5个字母，而每段之间不空行。第二种方法是空行不空格，即每段段首不空格，但段与段之间空一行。应该注意的是，这两种格式不能混用，即在同一篇文章中不可既有开头空格，又有段间空行。

(2) 关于逗号粘连错误(Comma Splice Error)

用逗号连接两个或两个以上完整的英文句子，这便构成了逗号粘连错误。逗号的使用在汉语和英语中区别很大。在汉语中，我们可以用逗号分隔两个句子，如："大学一年级学生的平均年龄是18岁或19岁，有些人小一两岁。"但在英语中，我们不能用逗号将这两个句子隔开：The average age of a college freshman is 18 or 19, some may be a year or two younger. 我们必须使用分号、破折号或句号。

(3) 关于A, B, and C模式

写作中我们常会罗列三个或三个以上的人或事物，这时应遵循的规范模式是A, B, and C。如：The little girl likes to sing, to dance, and to act. 这里要注意的是，and前的逗号不可少。有些英美作者会省去and前的逗号，这在有些语境中会引起歧义。如：He appealed to the administrators, the deans, and the chairmen。此句and前用了逗号，句中He呼吁的三种人很清楚，即the administrators, the deans和the chairmen；若不用最后的逗号，则He呼吁的人就可能是一种，即the administrators，因the deans and the chairmen可以是the administrators的同位语。

医护英语水平考试（二级）

模拟训练（一）

Medical English Test System（METS）Level 2

Ⅰ Listening

Part One

Questions 1—5

- You will hear five patients describing their problems. Decide what problem each patient has.
- Write the appropriate letter **A**—**H** in each box.
- Mark the corresponding letter on your **answer sheet**.
- You will hear each conversation twice.

Example:

0. Patient [F]

---

1. Patient 1 [ ]

2. Patient 2 [ ]

3. Patient 3 [ ]

4. Patient 4 [ ]

5. Patient 5 [ ]

A. Diabetes.

B. Arthritis.

C. Wound.

D. Anemia.

E. Pneumonia.

F. Stomachache.

G. Insomnia.

H. Influenza.

Part Two

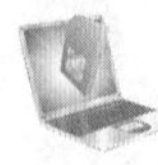

Questions 6—10

- You will hear a conversation between a patient and a nurse about health problem.
- For each of the following sentences, decide whether it is **True** (**A**) or **False** (**B**).

Put a tick (√) in the relevant box.
- Mark the corresponding letter on your **answer sheet**.
- You will hear the conversation twice.

Example:

0. The patient has a pain in the abdomen.
A. True ☑
B. False ☐

---

6. At first the patient had a pain in his stomach.
A. True ☐
B. False ☐

7. The patient has had vomiting for hours.
A. True ☐
B. False ☐

8. The nurse took the patient's temperature and found that there was a slight fever.
A. True ☐
B. False ☐

9. The patient was at ease all the time when having his abdomen checked.
A. True ☐
B. False ☐

10. The patient has appendicitis and will have an operation.
A. True ☐
B. False ☐

Part Three

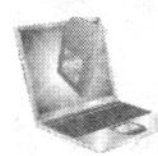

Questions 11—15

- You will hear a conversation between a patient and a doctor about Traditional Chinese Medicine (TCM).
- For each of the following questions or unfinished sentences, choose the correct answer **A**, **B** or **C**. Put a tick (√) in the relevant box.
- Mark the corresponding letter on your **answer sheet**.
- You will hear the conversation twice.

11. How does Mr. Smith think about acupuncture?

A. It is dissatisfying. ☐
B. It is really great. ☐
C. It is puzzling. ☐

12. In the TCM theory, the occurrence of diseases results from the incoordination between ________.

A. Yin and Yang ☐
B. body and mind ☐
C. diagnosis and treatment ☐

13. According to TCM, the treatment of diseases is ________.

A. to discover Yin and Yang ☐
B. to create Yin and Yang ☐
C. to restore the balance between Yin and Yang ☐

14. Which is right about the relationships between Yin and Yang?

A. They are always in harmony. ☐
B. They are contradictory. ☐
C. They never coordinate. ☐

15. Compared with Western medicine, what is the advantage of TCM in treating nervous system diseases?

A. Causing no pain. ☐
B. Leading to an earlier recovery. ☐
C. Causing no side effects. ☐

Part Four

Questions 16—20

- You will hear a conversation between a doctor and a patient about the treatment of wound.
- Fill in the blanks.
- Write the answers on your **answer sheet.**
- You will hear the conversation twice.

Surname (**16**) ________
Age 42 Sex M Marital Status M
Occupation Salesman
What Happened? The patient (**17**) ________, banging his head quite hard. The patient's wife (**18**)________ around the wound to stop the bleeding.
Treatment The patient will be given (**19**)________ for suture of the wound. The patient will have another (**20**) ________ injection since he has had it only once five years ago.
Points to Note Come again in 3 days for re-examination.

Ⅲ Reading and Writing

Part One

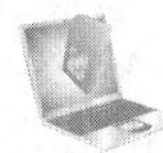

Questions 21—30

- Read the descriptions of the influence of attitude.
- Decide which part (**A**—**F**) mentions this (**21**—**30**). Some parts may be chosen more than once. Sentence **0** is an example.
- For each of the following questions, choose the correct answer **A**—**F**. Write the answer in the relevant box.
- Mark the corresponding letter on your **answer sheet**.

Which part(s) mention(s) that

- positive patients do better than those whose attitude is negative? **0** A
- self-affirming thoughts lead us to believe we will do well in the future? **21** ____

- negative attitude can interrupt the natural growth process? **22** ☐
- optimistic people outperform those who are doubtful? **23** ☐
- when we fail, we make a mental note to avoid similar situations in the future? **24** ☐
- the authority figures often shape our early thoughts? **25** ☐
- we play out the negative conditioning without thinking about it? **26** ☐
- learning to see yourself as a winner results from having successful experiences? **27** ☐
- small children's thoughts and feelings tend to be shaped by the authority figures? **28** ☐
- we remove ourselves from anxiety-producing situations? **29** ☐
- when we believe our efforts will be successful, we are more likely to undertake an activity? **30** ☐

A

We have noticed that patients who are positive about their recovery do better than those whose attitude is negative. In a broader sense, people with an optimistic view of themselves outperform those who are doubtful or simply more "realistic", even though their abilities are virtually identical. They don't give up easily or worry about obstacles because the final outcome is never in doubt—they see themselves as creative, resourceful problem solvers.

B

Why do some people see themselves as winners and act accordingly, while so many others don't? Learning to see yourself as a winner and to feel like a winner happens primarily as a result of having successful experiences and thinking self-affirming thoughts. When we believe our efforts will be successful, we are more likely to undertake an activity or task. Because we expect to succeed, we persist until we do.

C

This successful experience causes self-affirming thoughts, which boost our self-esteem, make us feel good, and lead us to believe we will do well in the future. Thus, we attempt more, and the upward spiral continues. This internal system helps us grow and develop—a natural continuous quality improvement program.

D

This is, however, an equally powerful downward spiral that can interrupt the natural growth process. If we believe we are likely to fail, we undertake activities tentatively, expecting a negative outcome. We feel anxious about our performance and we avoid or remove ourselves from anxiety-producing situations. When we fail, we say "I told you so" to ourselves and make a mental note to avoid similar situations in the future.

E

When we're very young, we have little to say about the experience to which we're subjected or the messages we receive from the world. The authority figures in our lives often shape our early thoughts and feelings. If they abuse this power, we may be conditioned to believe that the world is not a friendly place, that we have to struggle to get our basic needs met.

F

Years pass and the pattern repeats itself many times. It becomes part of who we are. We play out the negative conditioning without thinking about it.

Part Two

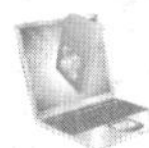

Questions 31—40

- Read the following passage.
- For each of the following sentences, decide whether it is **True** (**A**) or **False** (**B**). If there is not enough information to answer **True** (**A**) or **False** (**B**), choose **Not Given** (**C**).
- Mark the corresponding letter on your **answer sheet**.

Using Your Brain

If you want to stay young, sit down and have a good think. This is the research finding of a team of Japanese doctors, who say that most of our brains are not getting enough exercise—and as a result, we are aging unnecessarily soon.

Professor Taiju Matsuzawa wanted to find out why otherwise healthy farmers in northern Japan appeared to be losing their ability to think and reason at a relatively early age, and how the process of aging could be slowed down.

With a team of colleagues at Tokyo National University, he set about measuring brain volumes of a thousand people of different ages and various occupations.

Computer technology enabled the researchers to obtain precise measurements of the volume of the front and side sections of the brain, which are related to intellect and emotion and determine the human character. (The rear section of the brain, which controls functions like eating and breathing, does not contract with age, and one can continue living without intellectual or emotional faculties.)

Contraction of front and side parts—as cells die off—was observed in some subjects in their thirties, but it was still not evident in some sixty- and seventy-year-olds.

Matsuzawa concluded from his tests that there is a simple remedy to the contraction normally associated with age—using the brain.

The findings show in general terms that contraction of the brain begins sooner in people in the country than in the town. Those least at risk, says Matsuzawa, are lawyers, followed by university professors and doctors. White collar workers doing routine work in government offices are, however, as likely to have shrinking brains as farm workers, bus drivers and shop assistants.

Matsuzawa's findings show that thinking can prevent the brain from shrinking. Blood must circulate properly in the head to supply the fresh oxygen the brain cells need. "The best way to maintain good blood circulation is through using the brain," he says. "Think hard and engage in conversation. Don't rely on pocket calculators."

31. The team of doctors wanted to find out why certain people age sooner than others.

A. True **B.** False **C.** Not Given

32. Their research findings were based on the tests in one thousand old people.

A. True **B.** False **C.** Not Given

33. The doctor observed that the front section of the brain did not shrink in those people in their thirties.

A. True **B.** False **C.** Not Given

34. In the research, evident contraction of front and side parts was observed in all the subjects.

A. True **B.** False **C.** Not Given

35. According to the passage, lawyers seem to age faster than the others.

A. True **B.** False **C.** Not Given

36. According to the passage, the rear section of the brain does not contract with age.

A. True **B.** False **C.** Not Given

37. The front and side sections of the brain are related to intellect and emotion.

A. True **B.** False **C.** Not Given

38. White collar workers don't have shrinking brains.

A. True **B.** False **C.** Not Given

39. In general, contraction of the brain begins sooner in people in the town than in the country.

A. True **B.** False **C.** Not Given

40. The only remedy to the contraction is using the brain.

A. True **B.** False **C.** Not Given

Part Three

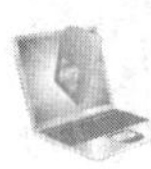

Questions 41—45

- Read the following passage.
- Choose the best answer **A**, **B** or **C**.
- Mark the corresponding letter on your **answer sheet**.

Death

People in the past did not question the difference between life and death. They could see that a person died when his heart stopped beating. People have learned, however, that the body does not die immediately when the heart stops beating. They discovered that we remain alive as long as our brain remains active. Today the difference between life and death is not as easy to see as in the past. Modern medical devices can keep the heart beating and the lungs breathing long after the brain stops. But is this life?

This question has caused much debate among citizens in the United States. Many of them want a law that says a person is dead when the brain dies. A person should be considered dead when brain waves stop even if machines can keep the body alive. Such a law would permit doctors to speed removal of healthy organs for transplant operations.

The brain is made of thousands of millions of nerve cells. These cells send and receive millions of chemical and electrical messages every day. In this way the brain controls the other body activities. Nerve-cell experts say that usually it is easy to tell when the brain has died. They put small electrodes(电极) on a person's skull to measure the electrical signals that pass in and out of the brain. These brain waves are recorded on a television screen or on paper. The waves move up and down every time the brain receives messages from the nerve cells. The brain is dead when the waves stop moving.

Although there are people who oppose the idea of a law on brain block for various reasons, the idea of brain wave activity as a test of death is slowly being accepted.

41. People in the past held that the difference between life and death ________.

A. was easy to tell **B.** did not exist **C.** lay in the brain

42. Which of the following is not true according to the passage?

A. The heart may keep beating after the brain has died.

B. The body dies immediately when the heart stops beating.

C. The brain may still be active after the heart has stopped beating.

43. When a person should be considered dead is currently a matter ________.

A. which has caused heated argument in the US
B. which few people in the US care much about
C. which only doctors can settle

44. The brain controls the other body activities through ________.
A. medical devices
B. small electrodes
C. the nerve cells

45. Gradually more and more people begin to accept the idea that a person is dead ________.
A. when the heart stops beating
B. when the brain becomes less active
C. when the brain stops working

Part Four >>>>>>

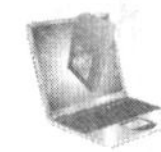

Questions 46—50

- Read the following procedures for dealing with minor cuts.
- Fill in each blank with the most appropriate procedure **A—F.** There is one extra procedure which you **DO NOT** need to use.
- Mark the corresponding letter on your **answer sheet.**

Procedures for Dealing with Minor Cuts

Ⅰ. Even minor cuts can become infected if they are left untreated. Any break in the skin can let bacteria enter the body.

Ⅱ. An increasing number of bacterial skin infections are resistant to antibiotic medicines. These infections can spread throughout the body. But taking good care of any injury that breaks the skin can help prevent an infection.

Ⅲ. Medical experts say the first step in treating a wound is to use clean water. Lake or ocean water should not be used.

Ⅳ. **(46)** ________.

Ⅴ. It is important to remove all dirt and other material from the wound.

Ⅵ. **(47)** ________.

Ⅶ. Studies have shown that these medicated products can help the healing.

Ⅷ. **(48)** ________.

Ⅸ. Finally, cover the cut with a clean bandage while it heals.

Ⅹ. **(49)** ________.

Ⅺ. As the wound heals, inspect for signs of infection including increased pain, redness and fluid around the cut.

Ⅻ. (**50**) ________.

XⅢ. If a wound seems infected, let the victim rest. Physical activity can spread the infection. If there are signs of infection, seek help from doctors or other skilled medical providers.

A. Change the bandage daily and keep the wound clean.
B. A high body temperature is also a sign of infection.
C. After the wound is cleaned, use a small amount of antibiotic ointment or cream.
D. They also help to keep the surface of the wound from becoming dry.
E. For larger wounds or in case bleeding does not stop quickly, use direct pressure. Place a clean piece of cloth on the area and hold it firmly in place until the bleeding stops or medical help arrives.
F. To clean the area around the wound, experts suggest using a clean cloth and soap. They say there is no need to use products like hydrogen peroxide or iodine.

Part Five

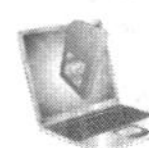

Questions 51—60

- Read the following passage.
- Choose the correct word for each blank from the list of words **A—L** given in the box below.
- Mark the corresponding letter on your **answer sheet**.

The First Line of Defense Against Germs

Think about all of the things that you touched today — from the telephone to the toilet. Whatever you did, you came into contact with germs and it's easy for germs on your hand to end up in your mouth.

Hand washing is a powerful way to (**51**) ________ the spread of disease.

Millions of lives could be saved each year if people washed their hands with soap often. Hand washing with soap could be among the most (**52**) ________ ways to reduce (**53**) ________ diseases.

Hand washing destroys germs from other people, animals or objects a person has touched. When people get (**54**) ________ on their hands, they can infect themselves by touching their eyes, nose or mouth. It's especially easy for a germ on your hand to end up in your mouth. Think about how much food you eat with your hands. But the worst thing is these people can infect other people. For example, the easiest way to catch cold is to touch your nose or eyes after someone nearby has (**55**) ________ or coughed. Another way to become sick is to eat food (**56**) ________ by someone whose hands were not clean. It is especially a good idea to wash your hands after (**57**) ________ money.

Good hand washing is your first line of (**58**) ________ against the (**59**) ________ of many illnesses—and not just the common cold. So never forget to (**60**) ________ your hands with water and dry them.

A. spread	**B.** defense	**C.** bacteria	**D.** effective
E. prevent	**F.** disease	**G.** infectious	**H.** touching
I. prepared	**J.** rinse	**K.** diagnose	**L.** sneezed

Part Six

Questions 61

- Read the patient admission form below.
- Use the information to write a case report of **no less than 100 words.**
- Write the report on your **answer sheet.**

Patient Admission Form

Patient: James Brown　　Age: 26 months
Gender: male　　Date of Admission: July 5, 2014

Chief Complaint:
- crying for 2 days

Signs and Symptoms:
- T: 41.2 ℃
- rash on neck and shoulders
- excessive mucus in nose and throat
- having difficulty in breathing
- vomit once every another hour

Diagnosis:
Dehydration

Nursing Instructions:
- drink much water
- be given a lukewarm sponge bath
- wear light bedclothes during daytime

医护英语水平考试（二级）

模拟训练（二）

Medical English Test System（METS）Level 2

I Listening

Part One >>>>>>

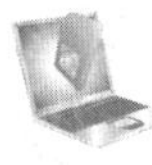

Questions 1—5

- You will hear five patients describing their problems. Decide what problem each patient has.
- Write the appropriate letter **A—H** in each box.
- Mark the corresponding letter on your **answer sheet.**
- You will hear each conversation twice.

Example:

0. Patient [F]

1. Patient 1 [ ]

2. Patient 2 [ ]

3. Patient 3 [ ]

4. Patient 4 [ ]

5. Patient 5 [ ]

A. Dizzy.
B. Fatigue.
C. Bruise.
D. Measles.
E. Influenza.
F. Stomachache.
G. Insomnia.
H. Infection.

Part Two >>>>>>

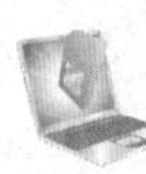

Questions 6—10

- You will hear a conversation between a patient and a nurse before an operation.
- For each of the following sentences, decide whether it is **True (A)** or **False (B)**. Put a tick (√) in the relevant box.
- Mark the corresponding letter on your **answer sheet.**

- You will hear the conversation twice.

Example:

0. The nurse checks the details relating to the operation.	**A.** True	✓
	B. False	

6. It's the first time the nurse has gone through the checklist for the patient.	**A.** True	
	B. False	
7. The patient will have a tendon repair operation in his left shoulder.	**A.** True	
	B. False	
8. The patient has not signed the consent form for the operation.	**A.** True	
	B. False	
9. The patient has just been given an injection before Wendy came.	**A.** True	
	B. False	
10. The nurse checks the identification and the bed number of the patient.	**A.** True	
	B. False	

Part Three

Questions 11—15

- You will hear a conversation between Patrica, a doctor, and Paul, a patient, about his discomforts.
- For each of the following questions or unfinished sentences, choose the correct answer **A**, **B** or **C**. Put a tick (√) in the relevant box.
- Mark the corresponding letter on your **answer sheet**.
- You will hear the conversation twice.

11. Where are Paul's pains?	**A.** In the cheek and the head.	
	B. In the arms and the chest.	
	C. Both A and B.	

12. How does Paul describe his pain in the shallow cuts?

A. Throbbing pain. ☐

B. Stinging pain. ☐

C. Sharp pain. ☐

13. How does Paul rate his pain when he is at rest?

A. At around six. ☐

B. At more than seven. ☐

C. At nearly ten. ☐

14. When does Paul's pain get worse?

A. When he moves. ☐

B. When he lies in bed. ☐

C. When he talks. ☐

15. What does the doctor do to relieve the patient's pain?

A. Pull the curtains around. ☐

B. Dim the lights. ☐

C. Give painkillers and a heat pack. ☐

Part Four

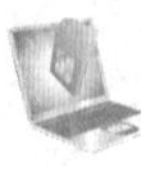

Questions 16—20

- You will hear a conversation between a doctor and a patient in the outpatient department.
- Fill in the blanks.
- Write the answers on your **answer sheet.**
- You will hear the conversation twice.

Surname Connolly	First Name Wentworth
Age (**16**) ________ Date of Admission April 3	Sex M Marital Status M
Hospital No. 453789	Expected Length of Stay (**17**) ________ Occupation (**18**) ________
Present Complaint (**19**)________ in the urine high blood pressure	

General Condition good
Pulse 70/min
Blood pressure (**20**) ________
Reason for Admission nephritis

Ⅱ Reading and Writing

Part One >>>>>>

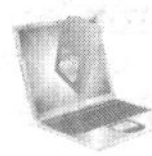

Questions 21—30

- Read the descriptions of several disorders and diseases.
- Decide which part (**A**—**F**) mentions this (**21**—**30**). Some parts may be chosen more than once. Sentence **0** is an example.
- For each of the following questions, choose the correct answer **A**—**F**. Write the answer in the relevant box.
- Mark the corresponding letter on your **answer sheet**.

Which part(s) mention(s) that

- massage and medicines are the common therapy? **0** E
- the main symptoms are skin rash, itching and asthma? **21** ____
- the inflamed organ needs to be removed by surgical operation? **22** ____
- the cause may involve damage to muscle and connective tissues? **23** ____
- it is an overreaction of the immune system? **24** ____
- the most common type is iron-deficiency anemia? **25** ____
- the pain begins in the naval area and then shifts to the lower right abdomen? **26** ____
- the general symptoms include fatigue, palpitation and shortness of breath? **27** ____
- the problem can be corrected by proper rest and nutrition? **28** ____

- the pain may also be accompanied by fever, nausea, vomiting and appetite loss? 29
- it is characterized by constant high levels of blood glucose? 30

A

Anemia is defined as a decrease in the amount of hemoglobin in the blood. It may result from too few red blood cells, cells that are too small, or too little hemoglobin in the cells. The general symptoms include fatigue, shortness of breath, heart palpitation and irritability. The most common type of anemia is iron-deficiency anemia caused by a lack of iron, which is required for hemoglobin production.

B

It is a harmful overreaction by the immune system, commonly known as allergy. In this case, a person is more sensitive to a particular antigen than the average individual. Common allergens are pollen, dust and foods, but there are many more. Responses may include itching, redness or tearing of the eyes, skin rash, asthma, sneezing, and urticaria(荨麻疹). An anaphylactic (过敏的) reaction is a severe generalized allergic response that can lead rapidly to death as a result of shock and interference with breathing.

C

Appendicitis occurs in all age groups, but is most common between the ages of 5 and 30. Symptoms typically begin with discomfort in the naval area that shifts into a steady, sharp pain in the lower right abdomen. A lower-grade fever may be present along with nauseated vomiting and loss of appetite. An inflamed appendix is usually surgically removed—delay in treatment may cause the appendix to rupture, resulting in peritonitis (infection of the abdominal cavity).

D

Muscle soreness is one of the common muscle disorders. It is often caused by hard muscular work. In severe cases, the soreness may last up to four days. The cause of muscle soreness is not completely understood, but it probably involves damage to muscle and connective tissue. With proper exercise, the muscles and body can adapt to strenuous muscle work and greatly reduce the risk of tissue damage.

E

Cramps occur when the normal operation of muscles is disturbed. Skeletal muscle cramps involve sudden and violent spastic(痉挛的) muscle contractions. No one knows exactly why such cramps occur. Cramps probably result from having too much or too little salt in the fluids surrounding muscle fibers. With proper rest and nutrition, the body can correct the problem, and cramping stops. Doctors use heat, massage and medicines in treating cramps.

F

Diabetes is a metabolic disorder where the human body does not produce or properly uses insulin, a hormone that is required to convert sugar, starches, and other food into energy. It's characterized by constant high levels of blood glucose (sugar). The human body has to maintain the blood glucose level at a very narrow range, which is done with insulin and glucagon(胰高血糖素).

Part Two >>>>>>

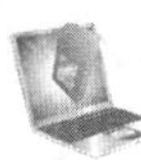

Questions 31—40

- Read the following passage.
- For each of the following sentences, decide whether it is **True** (**A**) or **False** (**B**). If there is not enough information to answer **True** (**A**) or **False** (**B**), choose **Not Given** (**C**).
- Mark the corresponding letter on your **answer sheet**.

Acute Gastroenteritis

Acute gastroenteritis could be more simply called a long and potentially lethal bout of stomach flu. The most common symptoms are diarrhea, vomiting and stomach pain, because whatever causes the condition inflames the gastrointestinal tract. Acute gastroenteritis is quite common among children, though it is certainly possible for adults to suffer from it as well. While most cases of gastroenteritis last a few days, acute gastroenteritis can last for weeks and months.

Numerous things may cause acute gastroenteritis. Bacterial infection is frequently a factor, and infection by parasites can cause acute gastroenteritis to last for several weeks. Viruses can also cause lengthy stomach flu. Accidental poisoning or exposure to toxins may also instigate acute gastroenteritis as well.

When a person does not recover from stomach flu symptoms within a day or so, it is usually a good idea to see a doctor. Some types of acute gastroenteritis will not resolve without antibiotic treatment, especially when bacteria or exposure to parasites are the cause. Physicians may want to diagnose the cause by analyzing a stool sample, when stomach symptoms remain problematic.

Another reason to seek medical treatment is that some forms of acute gastroenteritis mimic appendicitis, which may require emergency treatment. As well, young children run an especially high risk of becoming dehydrated during a long course of the stomach flu.

One should receive directions regarding how to help affected kids or adults get more fluids. Sometimes children, those with compromised immune systems, and the elderly may require hospitalization and intravenous fluids. Dehydration can actually cause greater nausea, and even organ shutdown if not properly addressed.

Even though causes for acute gastroenteritis vary, methods of transmission from one person to another usually remain the same. Generally, contact with the fecal matter of a person with the condition and then improperly washing or not washing the hands causes acute gastroenteritis to be quite contagious. Proper hand washing for both the ill person and well people in the family is always encouraged.

Other methods of transmission of acute gastroenteritis can include eating food or drinking liquids contaminated with bacteria or parasites. For example, poorly cooked hamburger might result in a very severe case of acute gastroenteritis due to exposure to E. coli, a sometimes lethal bacterial infection in young children.

31. The common symptoms of acute gastroenteritis are vomiting, diarrhea and stomach pain.

A. True **B.** False **C.** Not Given

32. Acute gastroenteritis is a disease that affects the gastrointestinal tract.

A. True **B.** False **C.** Not Given

33. Bacteria, viruses as well as parasites can lead to gastroenteritis.

A. True **B.** False **C.** Not Given

34. "Parasite" mentioned in the 2nd paragraph is a kind of bacteria.

A. True **B.** False **C.** Not Given

35. All types of gastroenteritis need to be treated with antibiotics after stool analysis.

A. True **B.** False **C.** Not Given

36. If the patient with acute gastroenteritis doesn't suffer from dehydration, it's not necessary to receive intravenous infusion.

A. True **B.** False **C.** Not Given

37. Dehydration is very dangerous because it may cause failure of many organs.

A. True **B.** False **C.** Not Given

38. The transmission route of acute gastroenteritis is not clear at present.

A. True **B.** False **C.** Not Given

39. Washing hands after each bowel movement can avoid transmission of acute gastroenteritis effectively.

A. True **B.** False **C.** Not Given

40. Eating and drinking something that has been contaminated with bacteria or parasites cannot increase the risk of gastroenteritis.

A. True **B.** False **C.** Not Given

Part Three >>>>>>

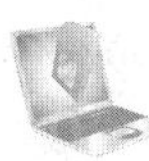

Questions 41—45

- Read the following passage.
- Choose the best answer **A**, **B** or **C**.
- Mark the corresponding letter on your **answer sheet**.

Cesarean Section

Not every woman undergoes a traditional vaginal delivery with the birth of her child. Under conditions of fetal distress, or in the case of breech presentation (when a baby is turned feet at the time of delivery), or if the woman's first baby was born by Cesarean delivery, a procedure called a Cesarean section may be required. A Cesarean section (often C-section, also other spellings) is a surgical procedure in which one or more incisions are made through a mother's abdomen (laparotomy) and uterus (hysterotomy) to deliver one or more babies, or, rarely, to remove a dead fetus. A Cesarean section is often performed when a vaginal delivery would put the baby's or mother's life or health at risk. Many are also performed upon request.

During a Cesarean section, a doctor will make either a lateral incision in the skin just above the pubic hair line, or a vertical incision below the naval. As the incision is made, blood vessels are cauterized to slow bleeding. After cutting through the skin, fat, and muscle of the abdomen, the membrane that covers the internal organs is opened, exposing the bladder and uterus. At this time the physician will generally insert his or her hands into the pelvis in order to determine the position of the baby and the placenta. Next, an incision is made into the uterus and any remaining fluids are suctioned from the uterus. The doctor then enlarges the incision with his or her fingers. The baby's head is then grasped and gently pulled with the rest of its body from the mother's uterus.

Finally, the abdominal layers are sewn together in the reverse order that they were cut. The mother is allowed to recover for approximately three to five days in the hospital. Typically, the recovery time depends on the patient and her pain tolerance and inflammation levels. She will be restricted from activity for the following several weeks.

There are several potential complications associated with this procedure that should be discussed with a doctor prior to surgery.

41. After cutting through the skin, fat, and muscle of the abdomen, the ________ that covers the internal organs is opened, exposing the bladder and uterus.

A. skin　　**B.** dermis　　**C.** membrane

42. As is mentioned in the text, after the procedure, the mother is allowed to recover for about ________ days in the hospital.

A. one to three **B.** two to five **C.** three to five

43. According to the passage, which condition doesn't require a Cesarean section?

A. The baby is turned feet when delivery.

B. The woman's first baby was born naturally.

C. The woman prefers to have a Cesarean section.

44. What is the position where a lateral incision is made?

A. In the skin above the pubic hair.

B. In the skin below the naval.

C. In the skin around the naval.

45. Which of the following statements is true according to the text?

A. There is more than one type of incision a doctor can choose to make in a Cesarean section.

B. When the bladder and uterus are exposed, the physician will rarely insert his or her hands into the pelvis.

C. At the end of a Cesarean, the abdominal layers are sewn together in the order that they were cut.

Part Four >>>>>>

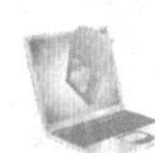

Questions 46—50

- Read the following procedures for administering IV infusion.
- Fill in each blank with the most appropriate procedure **A—F.** There is one extra procedure which you **DO NOT** need to use.
- Mark the corresponding letter on your **answer sheet.**

Procedures for Administering IV Infusion

Ⅰ. Get the IV bag ready.

Ⅱ. Before you start, please wash your hands.

Ⅲ. **(46)** ________

Ⅳ. **(47)** ________

Ⅴ. The giving set has one end to go into the IV bag and the other end is for connection to the patient's cannula.

Ⅵ. Run the Ⅳ infusion through an Ⅳ infusion pump.

Ⅶ. **(48)** ________

Ⅷ. Start the infusion pump and the pump is just for running a test.

Ⅸ. (**49**) ________

Ⅹ. Then, start the infusion.

Ⅺ. (**50**) ________

A. Set the rate on the infusion pump.
B. Check the IV solution against the IV prescription.
C. To prime the line, you run the IV fluid through the IV tubing of the giving set.
D. Sign the IV Prescription and write up the IV infusion on the Fluid Balance Chart.
E. Connect the IV to the patient's cannula.
F. Put on the sterile gloves and take care not to touch the outside of the gloves.

Part Five

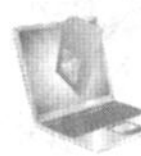

Questions 51—60

- Read the following passage.
- Choose the correct word for each blank from the list of words **A**—**L** given in the box below.
- Mark the corresponding letter on your **answer sheet**.

Source of Pain in Labor

The big question in everyone's mind is, "How much pain will there be for me during labor?" While we can't answer that question specifically, we can help (**51**) ________ some of the causes of pain and methods to deal with them.

There are three main causes of pain during childbirth: emotional, functional, and physiological.

Emotional sources of pain can be fear, the unknown, lack of education, etc. These can actually cause and intensify pain. Childbirth education is a great way to (**52**) ________ this problem, although it will not (**53**) ________ it. It will enable those participating in the birth process to have a working knowledge of what is going on. This is not limited to classroom instruction, but also (**54**) ________: reading, touring birth facility, discussion with care providers and numerous other sources of information.

Functional sources of pain can be cervical dilatation, contractions, descent of the baby, position, procedures, etc. Your muscles are (**55**) ________, and this may cause pain which can be reduced by relaxation. Holding your breath and fighting contractions can actually hinder dilatation and labor, and be more painful by (**56**) ________ your uterus of oxygen and creating tension. Position is very important in the birth process. Certain positions, such as (**57**) ________ on your back, can be harmful and painful. Changing positions and remaining (**58**) ________ can help to reduce this pain. Procedures, such as amniotomy(羊膜切开术), vaginal exams and monitoring can cause pain themselves, by limiting mobility, or by creating anxiety.

Physiological sources of pain will not (**59**) ________ with everyone, but are possibilities that you need to know how to deal with. One of the most common examples is a back labor caused by the posterior baby, this can occur in up to 25% of labors. This pain can be dealt with by trying to (**60**) ________ the baby to turn by using a variety of positions, water, etc. Sometimes unusual pain may be a sign of problems.

A. working	**B.** identify	**C.** mobile	**D.** depriving
E. discharge	**F.** encourage	**G.** produced	**H.** occur
I. includes	**J.** lying	**K.** eliminate	**L.** combat

Part Six

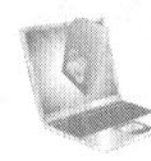

Questions 61

- Read the discharge summary below.
- Use the information to write a case report of **no less than 100 words**.
- Write the report on your **answer sheet**.

Discharge Summary
Patient: John Davis Age: 58 Sex: Male Date of Discharge: October 12, 2008 Date of Admission: October 7, 2008
Reason for admission: • A feeling of nausea. • Desire of vomiting. • A foreigner from UK, not get used to Chinese food.
Examination: • Bowel sounds in the examination of the abdomen.
Diagnosis: • Acute gastroenteritis; chronic non-atrophic(非萎缩性的) gastritis
Medication and Treatment: • Fluid rehydration and mineral supplement. • Antibiotics.
Prognosis and Needs: • No medications are needed after discharge. • Return to motherland if the patient still cannot get used to Chinese food. • Medical visit twice a month.

医护英语水平考试（二级）

模拟训练（三）

Medical English Test System（METS）Level 2

Ⅰ Listening

Part One >>>>>>

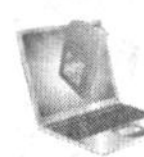

Questions 1—5

- You will hear five conversations about effects of some medications.
- What's the effect of each medication?
- For questions **1**—**5**, write a letter **A**—**G** next to each conversation.
- You will hear each conversation twice.

Example:

0. Medication 0 [F]

---

1. Medication 1 [ ]

2. Medication 2 [ ]

3. Medication 3 [ ]

4. Medication 4 [ ]

5. Medication 5 [ ]

A. To relieve pain.

B. To slow down aging.

C. To alleviate inflammation.

D. To reduce sputum production.

E. To slower the process of skin wrinkling.

F. To prevent bone diseases.

G. To balance body fluid.

Part Two >>>>>>

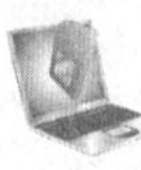

Questions 6—10

- You will hear a conversation between a patient and a nurse about his appendicitis.
- For each of the following sentences, decide whether it is **True** (**A**) or **False** (**B**). Put a tick (√) in the relevant box.
- Mark the corresponding letter on your **answer sheet**.
- You will hear the conversation twice.

Example:

0. The patient does not have a diarrhea. **A.** True ☑ **B.** False ☐

---

6. The patient has a pain in the abdomen. **A.** True ☐ **B.** False ☐

7. The patient has had vomiting for hours. **A.** True ☐ **B.** False ☐

8. The nurse took the patient's temperature and found that there was a slight fever. **A.** True ☐ **B.** False ☐

9. The patient was at ease when having his abdomen checked. **A.** True ☐ **B.** False ☐

10. The patient has appendicitis and will have an operation. **A.** True ☐ **B.** False ☐

Part Three

Questions 11—15

- You will hear a conversation between a patient and a doctor about treatment of eyes.
- For questions **11—15**, choose the correct answer **A**, **B** or **C**. Put a tick (√) in the box.
- You will hear the conversation twice.

---

11. The symptoms of the patient's eyes do not include ________.

A. pain ☐

B. being red ☐

C. abnormal eyesight ☐

12. The patient feels that ________.

A. there is secretion from his eyes ☐

B. his eyes fear light severely ☐

C. there is no itching in his eyes ☐

13. What should the patient do according to the doctor?

A. Put the eyedrops into his eyes twice per hour. ☐

B. Put the ointment into his eyes twice half an hour. ☐

C. There is no need for isolation. ☐

14. According to the doctor, the patient should not ________.

A. be sterilized regularly ☐

B. use hot compress ☐

C. wipe the eyes ☐

15. What will be helpful for the germs to develop and breed?

A. Not touching others' things. ☐

B. Not using hot compress. ☐

C. Covering the eyes. ☐

Part Four

Questions 16—20

- You will hear a doctor persuading a patient.
- Listen and complete questions **16**—**20** on your answer sheet.
- You will hear the conversation twice.

Name: (**16**) ________
Present Complaint The patient has got in her (**17**) ________ a lump of fibrosis (**18**) ________.
General Condition The tumor cannot be melted away by (**19**) ________ and an (**20**) ________ is the only way to stop the problem.
Points to Note Don't worry about hospitals.

Ⅱ Reading and Writing

Part One

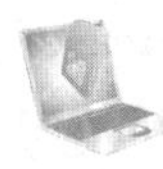

Questions 21—30

- Read the introduction about child maltreatment on the next page.
- Which case (**A**—**F**) mentions this (**21**—**30**)? The parts may be chosen more than once. There is an example at the beginning (**0**).
- Mark the correct letter **A**—**F** on your **answer sheet.**

Point out which part(s) mention(s)

• child treatment is a serious world wide problem.	0	A
• extreme stress can impair the development of the immune systems.	21	
• people have been identified several risk factors for child maltreatment.	22	
• there are no reliable global estimates for the prevalence of child maltreatment.	23	
• there is also an economic impact of child maltreatment.	24	
• a significant proportion of deaths are due to child maltreatment every year.	25	
• maltreatment causes stress associated with disruption in early brain development.	26	
• studies reveal that 25%—50% of all children report being physically abused.	27	
• every year, there are estimated 31,000 homicide deaths in children under 15.	28	
• maltreatment can lead to heart disease, cancer, suicide and sexually transmitted infections.	29	
• studies show that many children are subject to emotional abuse.	30	

A

Child maltreatment is a global problem with serious life-long consequences. There are no reliable global estimates for the prevalence of child maltreatment. Data for many countries, especially low-and-middle-income countries, are lacking.

B

Child maltreatment is complex and difficult to study. Current estimates vary widely depending on the country and the method of research used. Nonetheless, international studies reveal that approximately 20% of women and 5%—10% of men report being sexually abused as children, while 25%—50% of all children report being physically abused. Additionally, many children are subject to emotional abuse (sometimes referred to as psychological abuse).

C

Every year, there are estimated 31,000 homicide deaths in children under 15. This number underestimates the true extent of the problem, as a significant proportion of deaths due to child maltreatment are incorrectly attributed to falls, burns and drowning.

D

Child maltreatment causes suffering to children and families and can have long-term consequences. Maltreatment causes stress that is associated with disruption in early brain development. Extreme stress can impair the development of the nervous and immune systems. Consequently, as adults, maltreated children are at increased risk for behavioral, physical and mental health problems. Via the behavioral and mental health consequences, maltreatment can contribute to heart disease, cancer, suicide and sexually transmitted infections.

E

Beyond the health consequences of child maltreatment, there is an economic impact, including costs of hospitalization, mental health treatment, child welfare, and long-term health costs.

F

A number of risk factors for child maltreatment have been identified. These risk factors are not present in all social and cultural contexts, but provide an overview when attempting to understand the causes of child maltreatment.

Part Two >>>>>>

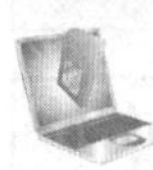

Questions 31—40

- Read the following passage.
- For each of the following sentences, decide whether it is **True (A)** or **False (B)**. If

there is not enough information to answer **True** (**A**) or **False** (**B**), choose **Not Given** (**C**).

- Mark the corresponding letter on your **answer sheet**.

Sun-Cure

Northern Europeans spend a lot of time in their cold and cloudy winters planning their summer holidays. They are proud of their healthy color when they return home after the holiday. But they also know that a certain amount of sunshine is good for their bodies and general health.

In ancient Greece people knew about the healing powers of the sun, but this knowledge was lost. At the end of the nineteenth century a Danish doctor, Niels Finsen, began to study the effect of sunlight on certain diseases, especially diseases of the skin. He was interested not only in natural sunlight but also in artificially produced rays. Sunlight began to play a more important part in curing sick people.

A Swiss doctor, Auguste Rollier, made full use of the sun in his hospital at Lysine. Lysine is a small village high up in the Alps. The position is important: the rays of the sun with the greatest healing power are the infra-red(红外线的) and ultra-violet(紫外线的) rays; but ultra-violet rays are too easily lost in fog and the polluted air near industrial towns. Dr. Roller found that sunlight, fresh air and good food cure a great many diseases. He was particularly successful in curing certain forms of tuberculosis with his "sun-cure". There were a large number of children in Dr. Roller's hospital. He decided to start a school where sick children could be cured and at the same time continue to learn. It was not long before his school was full. In winter, wearing only shorts, socks and boots, the children put on their skis after breakfast and left the hospital. They carried small desks and chairs as well as their school books. Their teacher led them over the snow until they reached a slope which faced the sun and was free from cold winds. There they set out their desks and chairs, and school began. Although they wore hardly any clothes, Roller's pupils were very seldom cold. That was because their bodies were full of energy which they got from the sun.

But the doctor knew that sunshine can also be dangerous. If, for example, tuberculosis is attacking the lungs, unwise sunbathing may do great harm. Today there is not just one school in the sun. There are several in Switzerland, and since Switzerland is not the only country which has the right conditions, there are similar schools in other places.

31. Northern Europeans know that a certain amount of sunshine is good for their general health.

A. True **B**. False **C**. Not Given

32. Ancient people knew nothing about the healing powers of the sun.

A. True **B**. False **C**. Not Given

33. People didn't use sunlight to cure sick people for a long time in history.

A. True **B**. False **C**. Not Given

34. Niels Finsen was interested not in natural sunlight but in artificially produced rays.

A. True **B**. False **C**. Not Given

35. If tuberculosis is attacking the lungs, unwise sunbathing may be very harmful.

A. True **B**. False **C**. Not Given

36. The rays of the sun with the greatest healing power are only the infra-red rays.

A. True **B**. False **C**. Not Given

37. Ultra-violet rays are too easily lost in fog and the polluted air.

A. True **B**. False **C**. Not Given

38. Amiable environment may help cure many diseases.

A. True **B**. False **C**. Not Given

39. Dr. Roller started a school in which sick children could be cured and continue to learn.

A. True **B**. False **C**. Not Given

40. Roller's pupils were seldom cold because they wore a lot.

A. True **B**. False **C**. Not Given

Part Three

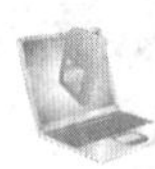

Questions 41—45

- Read the passage on obesity.
- For questions **41**—**45**, choose the answer (**A**, **B**, or **C**) which you think fits best according to the passage.
- Mark the correct letter **A**, **B**, or **C** on your **answer sheet**.

Obesity

Obesity means having too much body fat. It is different from being overweight, which means weighing too much. The weight may come from muscle, bone, fat and/ or body water. Both terms mean that a person's weight is greater than what's considered healthy for his or her height.

Obesity occurs over time when you eat more calories than you use. The balance between calories-in and calories-out differs for each person. Factors that might tip the balance include your genetic makeup, overeating, eating high-fat foods and not being physically active.

Data show that among adults aged 20-74 the prevalence of obesity increased from 15.0% in the 1976-1980 survey to 32.9% in the 2003-2004 survey.

The two surveys also show increases in obesity among children and teens. For children aged 2-5, the prevalence of obesity increased from 5.0% to 13.9%; for those aged 6-11, prevalence increased from 6.5% to 18.8%; and for those aged years, prevalence increased form 5.0% to 17.4%.

These increasing rates raise concern because of their implications for Americans' health. Being overweight or obese increases the risk of many diseases and health conditions, including: hypertension (high blood pressure), osteoarthritis(骨关节炎), dyslipidemia(血脂异常), type Ⅱ diabetes, coronary heart disease, stroke, gallbladder disease, sleep apnea and respiratory problems, some cancers(endometrial, breast, and colon).

If you are obese, losing even 5 to 10 percent of your weight can delay or prevent some of these diseases.

41. The weight may come from ________.

A. muscle and/or bone

B. fat and/or body water

C. All of the above

42. The following factors might tip the balance between calories-in and calories-out **EXCEPT** ________.

A. genetic makeup

B. working out properly

C. overeating

43. Among which population did the prevalence of obesity increase most according to the passage?

A. Children aged 6-11.

B. Teens aged 12-19.

C. Adults aged 20-74.

44. According to the passage, many diseases are caused by ________.

A. fast food

B. getting old

C. being obese

45. Which of the following statements is NOT true according to the passage?

A. If you lose even 5 to 10 percent of your weight, some disease can be delayed or prevented.

B. The prevalence of obesity is on a rise in America.

C. Obesity may result in breast cancer.

Part Four >>>>>>

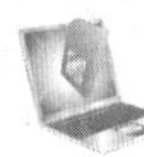

Questions 46—50

- Read the following procedures of heart transplantation.
- Choose from the procedures **A—F** the one which fits each gap (**46—50**). There is one extra procedure which you do not need to use.
- Mark your answers on the separate **answer sheet**.

Procedures for Heart Transplantation

Ⅰ. A typical heart transplantation begins when a suitable donor heart is identified.

Ⅱ. (**46**) ________, also called a beating heart cadaver.

Ⅲ. The patient is contacted by a nurse coordinator and instructed to come to the hospital for evaluation and pre-surgical medication.

Ⅳ. (**47**) ________.

Ⅴ. Learning that a potential organ is unsuitable can induce distress in an already fragile patient, who usually requires emotional support before returning home.

Ⅵ. (**48**) ________.

Ⅶ. The patient is also given immunosuppressant medication so that the patient's immune system does not reject the new heart.

Ⅷ. Once the donor heart passes inspection, the patient is taken into the operating room and given a general anaesthetic.

Ⅸ. After the operation, the patient is taken to the ICU to recover. (**49**) ________.

Ⅹ. The duration of in-hospital, post-transplant care depends on the patient's general health, how well the heart is working, and the patient's ability to look after the new heart.

Ⅺ. (**50**) ________.

Ⅻ. After release, the patient returns for regular check-ups and rehabilitation.

A. At the same time, the heart is removed from the donor and inspected by a team of surgeons to see if it is in suitable condition

B. When they wake up, they move to a special recovery unit for rehabilitation

C. The heart comes from a recently deceased or brain dead donor

D. Doctors typically prefer that patients leave the hospital 1-2 weeks after surgery, because of the risk of infection and presuming no complications

E. The frequency of hospital visits decreases as the patient adjusts to the transplant

F. The patient must also undergo emotional, psychological, and physical tests to verify mental health and ability to make good use of a new heart

Part Five >>>>>>

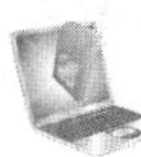

Questions 51—60

- Read the following passage.
- Choose the best word for each space from a list of choices (**A**—**L**) given in the box following the passage.
- For each space **51**—**60**, mark one letter **A**—**L** on your **answer sheet.**

Allergy

An allergy is a hypersensitivity disorder of the immune system. Symptoms include red eyes, itchiness, and runny nose, eczema, hives, or an asthma attack. The symptoms of allergy vary with allergen, and with the part of the body affected.

The (**51**) ________ or allergic reaction, may include sneezing, watery eyes, and nasal congestion, as in hay fever which selects an allergic rhinitis; a rash, stomach upset, and itchy swelling on the skin, as in some food or drugs that (**52**) ________ with breathing, as in asthma; and in rare anaphylactic shock, which may lead to choke and death. Anaphylactic shock occasionally follows injections of penicillin or other (**53**) ________ and may sometimes follow the sting of a bee or a wasp.

Allergic reactions occur when a person's (**54**) ________ system reacts to normally harmless substances in the environment. A substance that causes a reaction is called an (**55**) ________. These reactions are acquired, predictable, and rapid. Allergy is one of four forms of hypersensitivity and is formally called type Ⅰ (or immediate) hypersensitivity. Allergic reactions are distinctive because of excessive activation of certain white blood cells called mast cells and basophils by a type of antibody called immunoglobulin E (IgE). This reaction results in an (**56**) ________ response which can range from uncomfortable to dangerous.

A variety of tests exist to (**57**) ________ allergic conditions. If done they should be ordered and interpreted in light of a person's history of exposure as many (**58**) ________ test results do not mean a clinically significant allergy. Tests include placing possible allergens on the skin and looking for a (**59**) ________ such as swelling and blood tests to look for an allergen-specific IgE.

Treatments for (**60**) ________ include avoiding known allergens, steroids that modify the immune system in general, and medications such as antihistamines and decongestants which reduce symptoms.

A. allergen	B. positive	C. allergies	D. diagnose
E. reaction	F. inflammatory	G. drugs	H. immune
I. interfere	J. resist	K. symptoms	L. syndrome

Part Six

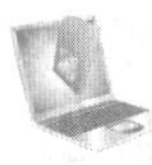

Questions 61

- Read the following patient's chart.
- Use the information to write a patient report.
- Write the report in about **100 words** on your **answer sheet.**

Patient's Chart	
Patient: John Gender: Male	Age: 26 DOA: 2014/04/03
Symptoms: • severe acute right upper abdominal pain • rigidity of abdominal muscle	
Chief Complaint: • hunger-like pain occurring at night or after meals • food is of no use to reduce the pain	
Examination: positive occult blood test and decreased CBC(complete blood count).	
Diagnosis: duodenal ulcer with perforation(十二指肠溃疡并发穿孔).	
Treatment and present condition: • operation • in good condition	
Needs: • enough rest and sleep • check-up in 20 days	

医护英语水平考试（二级）

模拟训练（四）

Medical English Test System（METS）Level 2

I Listening

Part One >>>>>>

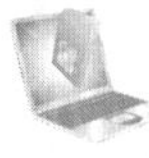

Questions 1—5

- You will hear five patients describing their problems. Decide what problem each patient has.
- Write the appropriate letter **A**—**H** in each box.
- Mark the corresponding letter on your **answer sheet.**
- You will hear each conversation twice.

Example:

0. Patient **D**

---

1. Patient 1 ☐

2. Patient 2 ☐

3. Patient 3 ☐

4. Patient 4 ☐

5. Patient 5 ☐

A. Diabetes.

B. Anemia.

C. Pneumonia.

D. Arthritis.

E. Appendicitis.

F. Headache.

G. Asthma.

H. Difficult swallowing.

Part Two >>>>>>

Questions 6—10

- You will hear a conversation between a patient and a nurse about the acute appendicitis.
- For each of the following sentences, decide whether it is **True** (**A**) or **False** (**B**).

Put a tick (√) in the relevant box.
- Mark the corresponding letter on your **answer sheet**.
- You will hear the conversation twice.

Example:

0. The woman had a terrible pain in her belly.
A. True ☑
B. False ☐

---

6. The woman had a stomachache for 3 days.
A. True ☐
B. False ☐

7. The woman had diarrhea just now.
A. True ☐
B. False ☐

8. The woman had a slight fever.
A. True ☐
B. False ☐

9. The blood test shows her white blood cell count.
A. True ☐
B. False ☐

10. The woman will have to take an operation.
A. True ☐
B. False ☐

Part Three

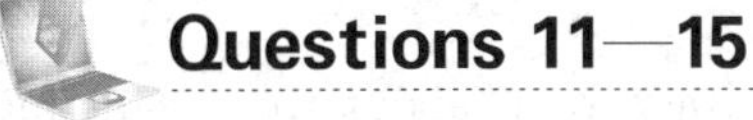

Questions 11—15

- You will hear a conversation between a patient and a nurse about post-operative care.
- For each of the following questions or unfinished sentences, choose the correct answer **A**, **B** or **C**. Put a tick (√) in the relevant box.
- Mark the corresponding letter on your **answer sheet**.
- You will hear the conversation twice.

11. Why did the nurse get the patient out of bed so early?

- **A.** It was meal time. ☐
- **B.** It can prevent complications. ☐
- **C.** It was the doctor's order. ☐

12. This is an incentive spirometer(肺活量测量计) which is to help the patient to ________.

- **A.** recover his wound ☐
- **B.** sleep quickly ☐
- **C.** breathe more deeply ☐

13. What does this machine help him to prevent?

- **A.** Headache. ☐
- **B.** Cancer. ☐
- **C.** Pneumonia. ☐

14. Why did the doctor listen to his abdomen?

- **A.** For bowel sounds. ☐
- **B.** For side effects. ☐
- **C.** For terrible pain. ☐

15. Why is the nurse keeping the patient up?

- **A.** It is her job. ☐
- **B.** It is her habit. ☐
- **C.** It is her joy. ☐

Part Four >>>>>>

Questions 16—20

- You will hear a conversation between a nurse and a patient about the meals and food.
- Fill in the blanks.
- Write the answers on your **answer sheet**.
- You will hear the conversation twice.

MEALS AND FOOD
Breakfast time (**16**) ________ AM Dinner time (**17**) ________ PM
Muslim: N/A
The preference for food kind: He likes (**18**) ________ food very much. His appetite is not good. He would like to have a snack in the afternoon and before going to bed.
Allergic food: (**19**) ________ food
He likes rice (**20**) ________. It's important for him to eat a little more.

Ⅱ Reading and Writing

Part One

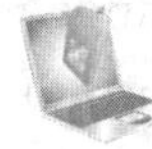

Questions 21—30

- Read the descriptions of some diseases.
- Decide which part (**A**—**F**) mentions this (**21**—**30**). Some parts may be chosen more than once. Sentence **0** is an example.
- For each of the following questions, choose the correct answer **A**—**F**. Write the answer in the relevant box.
- Mark the corresponding letter on your **answer sheet**.

Which part(s) mention(s) that

• the disease is flu, and the symptom can be mild and severe?	**0**	**A**
• there is a lot of pain in the abdomen?	**21**	
• the blood test tells that hemoglobin(血红蛋白) is low?	**22**	
• asthma is one of the risk factors?	**23**	

- the infection of this disease is progressive and may not be noticed? **24**
- the disease makes the patient feel like going to pass out? **25**
- the symptom like coughing may last over two weeks? **26**
- the patient's blood sugar level is high and has frequent urination? **27**
- chest X-ray, blood tests, and culture of the sputum help to confirm this disease? **28**
- a patient who has this disease may feel nausea and have bad appetite? **29**
- if the disease comes on quickly, it often has greater symptoms? **30**

A

It is an infectious disease caused by an influenza virus. Symptoms can be mild to severe. The most common symptoms include: a high fever, runny nose, sore throat, muscle pains, headache, coughing, and feeling tired. These symptoms typically begin two days after exposure to the virus and most last less than a week. The cough, however, may last for more than two weeks. In children, there may be nausea and vomiting, but these are not common in adults.

B

It is inflammation of the appendix (阑尾). Symptoms commonly include lower right abdominal pain, nausea, vomiting, and decreased appetite. However, approximately 40% of people do not have these typical symptoms. Severe complications of a ruptured appendix include widespread, painful inflammation of the inner lining of the abdominal wall and sepsis.

C

It is usually caused by infection with viruses or bacteria and less commonly by other microorganisms, certain medications and conditions such as autoimmune(自身免疫的) diseases. Risk factors include other lung diseases such as cystic fibrosis (囊性纤维变性), COPD, and asthma, diabetes, heart failure, a history of smoking, a poor ability to cough such as following a stroke, or a weak immune system. Diagnosis is often based on the symptoms and physical examination. Chest X-ray, blood tests, and culture of the sputum may help confirm the diagnosis.

D

It is a decrease in the total amount of red blood cells (RBCs) or hemoglobin(血红蛋白) in the blood, or a lowered ability of the blood to carry oxygen. When anemia comes on slowly, the symptoms are often vague and may include feeling tired, weakness, shortness of breath or a poor ability to exercise. Anemia that comes on quickly often has greater symptoms, which may include confusion, feeling like one is going to pass out, loss of consciousness, or increased thirst.

Anemia must be significant before a person becomes noticeably pale. Additional symptoms may occur depending on the underlying cause.

E

Following initial infection, a person may not notice any symptoms or may experience a brief period of influenza-like illness. Typically, this is followed by a prolonged period with no symptoms. As the infection progresses, it interferes more with the immune system, increasing the risk of common infections like tuberculosis.

F

It is a group of metabolic disorders in which there are high blood sugar levels over a prolonged period. Symptoms of high blood sugar include frequent urination, increased thirst, and hunger.

Part Two >>>>>>

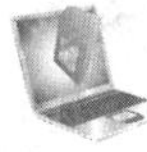

Questions 31—40

- Read the following passage.
- For each of the following sentences, decide whether it is **True (A)** or **False (B)**. If there is not enough information to answer **True (A)** or **False (B)**, choose **Not Given (C)**.
- Mark the corresponding letter on your **answer sheet**.

Sense of Smell

In addition to bringing out the flavor of food, what does the sense of smell do for us? Smell "gives us information about place, about where we are," says Randall Reed, a Johns Hopkins University professor whose specialty is the sense of smell. And smell tells us about people.

"Whether we realize it or not, we collect a lot of information about who is around us based on smell," says Reed. Even at a distance, odors can warn us of trouble—spoiled food, leaking gas, or fire. "It's a great alert," offers Donald Leopold, a doctor at Johns Hopkins. For example, if something in the oven is burning, everyone in the house knows it.

With just a simple scent, smell can also evoke very intense emotion. Let's say, for example, that the smell is purple petunias(喇叭花). These flowers have a rich emotions that no other petunia has. Now let's imagine that your mother died when you were three, and she used to have a flower garden. You wouldn't need to identify the smell or to have conscious memories of your mother or her garden. You would feel sad as soon as you smelled that spicy odor.

Compared with animals, how well do people detect smells? That depends on what you mean by "how well". We are low on receptor cells: current estimates say that humans have roughly five million smell-receptor cells, about as many as a mouse. A rat has some 10 million, a rabbit 20 million, and a bloodhound 100 million.

Reed says that, across species, there is a relatively good correlation between the number of receptor cells and how strong the sense of smell is. "You can hardly find the olfactory bulb in a human brain—it's a pea-sized object. In a mouse, it's a little bigger. It's bean-sized in a rat, about the size of your little finger in a rabbit, and the size of your thumb in a bloodhound."

31. Smell gives us information about place and people.
A. True **B.** False **C.** Not Given

32. Randall Reed is not a specialist in the sense of smell.
A. True **B.** False **C.** Not Given

33. Odors can help the police to detect criminal cases.
A. True **B.** False **C.** Not Given

34. At a distance, odors cannot warn us of trouble.
A. True **B.** False **C.** Not Given

35. The underlined word "alert" in Paragraph 3 means "on guard".
A. True **B.** False **C.** Not Given

36. According to the passage, if something in the oven is burning, everybody in the house will know it.
A. True **B.** False **C.** Not Given

37. It is impossible that smell can evoke very intense emotion.
A. True **B.** False **C.** Not Given

38. If your mother died when you were three, you would feel sad when you smell the odor which belongs to your mother's garden.
A. True **B.** False **C.** Not Given

39. Humans have fewer receptor cells than animals.
A. True **B.** False **C.** Not Given

40. The key to detecting smells depends on receptor cells.
A. True **B.** False **C.** Not Given

Part Three >>>>>>

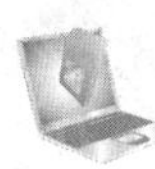

Questions 41—45

- Read the following passage.
- Choose the best answer **A**, **B** or **C**.
- Mark the corresponding letter on your **answer sheet**.

Allergy

Allergy has become more and more common over the last 30 years. Now one-third of us are affected by allergy at some point in our lives and half of these sufferers are children. In the UK, three million people suffer from asthma, and five per cent of children suffer from food allergy.

Allergy is a reaction that occurs when the immune system has a strange and unnecessary reaction to a substance which is normally harmless, such as pollen(花粉) or peanuts. The immune system is there to protect the body against outside attackers, including viruses, bacteria and parasites. To defend your body against an attacker, the immune system remembers these dangerous micro-organisms and attacks them if it meets them again. This work is done by antibodies. The immune system in allergy sufferers makes antibodies against harmless substances, because it mistakenly believes them to be dangerous.

An allergic reaction may not happen the first time a sufferer meets an allergen (the substance causing the reaction, such as pollen, milk or strawberries). Sometimes people can eat nuts for years and then suddenly become allergic to them. What has happened is that the immune system has now decided the substance is dangerous and has made an allergy antibody. This antibody then attaches itself to cells, which contain histamine(组胺). When the antibodies meet the allergen the next time, they try to destroy it. As they do that, the surface of the cells is broken, and histamine is released.

The histamine and other chemicals inflame the tissues. This leads to the symptoms of allergy, such as swelling, rashes, sneezing, sore eyes and breathlessness. Anaphylaxis(全身过敏性反应) is the most severe allergic reaction of all and is most often triggered by wasp or bee stings or peanuts. This must be treated immediately.

41. Allergy has become more and more common because ________.

A. one-third of us are affected by allergy in different periods

B. all of us have the experience of allergy

C. half of our children have allergy in the past 30 years

42. The immune system is there to protect the body against outside attackers, including ________.

A. genes, pollen, and virus

B. viruses, bacteria, and parasites

C. viruses, bacteria, and peanuts

43. The immune system in allergy sufferers makes antibodies because ________.

A. it mistakenly believes the immune system is dangerous

B. it mistakenly believes the allergic substances are dangerous

C. it mistakenly believes the harmless substances are dangerous

44. Sometimes people can eat nuts for years and then suddenly become allergic to them, because ________.

A. the immune system has now decided the substance is dangerous

B. the immune system has forgotten to produce antibodies

C. the immune system refused to work

45. Which of the following CANNOT be inferred from the passage?

A. We are safe because we are not attacked by the allergic substances.

B. Swelling is one of the symptoms of allergy.

C. Antibodies play important roles in the process of allergy.

Part Four >>>>>>

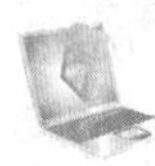

Questions 46—50

- Read the following procedures for preparing the treatment room.
- Fill in each blank with the most appropriate procedure **A—F.** There is one extra procedure which you **DO NOT** need to use.
- Mark the corresponding letter on your **answer sheet.**

Procedures for Preparing the Treatment Room

Ⅰ. Doctor Hehn is going to stitch Paul's cut and Anna is getting the treatment room ready. The procedures are as follows:

Ⅱ. Firstly, (**46**) ________ For this she needs a swab and a pair of tweezers.

Ⅲ. Next, (**47**) ________ For this she needs a syringe.

Ⅳ. Then (**48**) ________

Ⅴ. After that (**49**) ________

Ⅵ. Finally (**50**) ________
Ⅶ. A few days later she takes the stitches out.
Ⅷ. For this she needs a pair of scissors and a pair of tweezers.

A. she gives a local anaesthetic.
B. she stitches the wound with a needle and thread.
C. Dr. Hehn examines the patient and then cleans the wound.
D. she dresses the wound with a gauze dressing and a bandage.
E. press the wound in order to eliminate pus.
F. she ties off the stitches.

Part Five

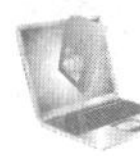

Questions 51—60

- Read the following passage.
- Choose the correct word for each blank from the list of words **A**—**L** given in the box below.
- Mark the corresponding letter on your **answer sheet**.

Leukemia(白血病)

Leukemia is the most common type of cancer kids get, but it is still very rare. Leukemia involves the blood and bloodforming (**51**) ________, such as the bone marrow.

Bone marrow is the innermost part of some bones where blood cells are first made. A kid with leukemia produces lots of (**52**) ________ white blood cells in the bone marrow. Usually, white blood cells (**53**) ________ infection, but the white blood cells in a person with leukemia don't work the way they're supposed to. They don't protect the person from (**54**) ________ very well.

The abnormal white blood cells multiply out of control, filling the bone marrow and making it hard for enough (**55**) ________, infection-fighting white blood cells to form. Other blood cells—such as red blood cells (that carry (**56**) ________ in the blood to the body's tissues) and platelets (that allow blood to clot)—are also crowded out by the (**57**) ________ blood cells of leukemia.

These cancer cells may also (**58**) ________ to other parts of the body, including the (**59**) ________, where they continue to multiply and build up. Although leukemia can make kids sick, most of the time it is (**60**) ________, and kids get better.

Almost all leukemia patients are treated with chemotherapy, which means using anti-cancer drugs.

A. fight	**B.** infections	**C.** normal	**D.** organs
E. move	**F.** abnormal	**G.** oxygen	**H.** white
I. treatable	**J.** dangerous	**K.** blood stream	**L.** body

Part Six

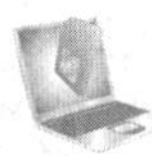

Questions 61

- Read the patient care plan below.
- Use the information to write a case report of **no less than 100 words.**
- Write the report on your **answer sheet.**

Patient Care Plan
Patient: Mr. Jason Hoover
Next of kin: Mr. Leo Hoover (son)
Needs/problems: Dehydration, inadequate fluid intake, dry and dehydrated skin. Dry lips, and coated tongue. Decreased urinary output.
Objectives: Adequate hydration. Moist lips & tongue. Urinary output of at least 2,000 ml per day.
Nursing interventions: Ensure fluid at least 3,000 ml daily. Sit the patient well before giving drinks. Offer drinks hourly (preferably tea/lemon, rather than coffee). Give mouth care 4-hourly. Observe & record output, report inadequate output.

医护英语水平考试(二级)

模拟训练(五)

Medical English Test System (METS) Level 2

I Listening

Part One >>>>>

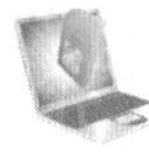

Questions 1—5

- You will hear five patients describing their problems. Decide what problem each patient has.
- Write the appropriate letter A—H in each box.
- Mark the corresponding letter on your **answer sheet**.
- You will hear each conversation twice.

Example:

0. Patient [E]

---

1. Patient 1 [ ]

2. Patient 2 [ ]

3. Patient 3 [ ]

4. Patient 4 [ ]

5. Patient 5 [ ]

A. Rash.
B. Loss of appetite.
C. Difficulty swallowing.
D. Asthma.
E. Arthritis.
F. Backache.
G. Diabetes.
H. Pneumonia.

Part Two >>>>>

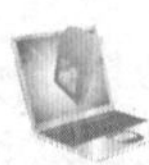

Questions 6—10

- You will hear a conversation between a patient and a nurse about the test results.
- For each of the following sentences, decide whether it is **True** (**A**) or **False** (**B**). Put a tick (√) in the relevant box.
- Mark the corresponding letter on your **answer sheet**.

- You will hear the conversation twice.

Example:

0. The woman did an ultrasound test. **A.** True ☑ **B.** False ☐

---

6. The woman had vomited for hours. **A.** True ☐ **B.** False ☐

7. The woman did an ultrasound test just now. **A.** True ☐ **B.** False ☐

8. The test results are very good. **A.** True ☐ **B.** False ☐

9. The woman felt satisfied when she heard the fetus position was a little low. **A.** True ☐ **B.** False ☐

10. This is a pregnant woman who did her prenatal care. **A.** True ☐ **B.** False ☐

Part Three

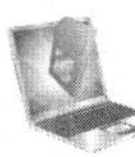

Questions 11—15

- You will hear a conversation between a patient and a nurse about pain.
- For each of the following questions or unfinished sentences, choose the correct answer **A**, **B** or **C**. Put a tick (√) in the relevant box.
- Mark the corresponding letter on your **answer sheet**.
- You will hear the conversation twice.

11. Where was Mr. Jameson's first pain?

A. Around his prostate(前列腺). ☐
B. On his left arm. ☐
C. On his left ankle. ☐

12. The first pain of Mr. Jameson was caused by ________.

A. his wound ☐
B. his joints ☐
C. his main cancer ☐

13. What made Mr. Jameson's first pain better?

A. A painkiller. ☐
B. A non-stick dressing. ☐
C. A syringe driver. ☐

14. Which scale did Mr. Jameson describe his second pain?

A. Six. ☐
B. Two. ☐
C. Six and two. ☐

15. When did the second pain especially hurt?

A. When he got out of the bed. ☐
B. When the dressing was changed. ☐
C. When he walked around. ☐

Part Four >>>>>>

Questions 16—20

- You will hear a conversation between a doctor and a patient about the discharge medication.
- Fill in the blanks.
- Write the answers on your **answer sheet.**
- You will hear the conversation twice.

Surname John Feldman		
AGE (**16**) ________	SEX M	**MARITAL STATUS** M
OCCUPATION Salesman		
The first medication This capsule is (**17**) ________. Make sure you take it on empty stomach and (**18**) ________ a day.		
The second medication These are your eye drops. They last only a month so remember to (**19**) ________ the contents after this date. They should be kept in the fridge.		
The third medication This is the lotion for your rash. It's important that you (**20**) ________ the bottle so you can mix the contents well.		

Ⅱ Reading and Writing

Part One

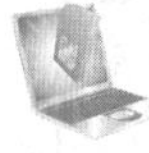

Questions 21—30

- Read the descriptions of preserving the organs.
- Decide which part (**A**—**F**) mentions this (**21**—**30**). Some parts may be chosen more than once. Sentence **0** is an example.
- For each of the following questions, choose the correct answer **A**—**F**. Write the answer in the relevant box.
- Mark the corresponding letter on your **answer sheet.**

Which part(s) mention(s) that

- heart can be damaged after 10 to 30 minutes without a blood supply? | **0** | **A** |

- it is unnecessary to use complicated ways to preserve the kidney? **21**
- to keep a kidney undamaged for 48—72 hours, we need a complicated machine to provide artificial circulation? **22**
- ice crystals can keep cells from getting worse but may have a bad effect on kidney? **23**
- the kidney on the donor can be moved to the receiver at once? **24**
- blood cells can be kept alive when frozen to subzero temperatures? **25**
- the kidney removed from the donor should be infused with cool fluid for preserving? **26**
- the brain is more delicate than most organs? **27**
- the kidney for transplanting should be kept without oxygen? **28**
- to keep a kidney useful more than 3 days is difficult? **29**
- to some degree, the cornea can be removed for grafting without hurrying? **30**

A

Without a blood supply organs deteriorate rapidly. Cooling can slow down the process but cannot stop it. Organs differ in their sensitivity to damage. At body temperature, permanent destruction of the brain occurs after more than three to five minutes; of the heart, liver, and lung, after 10 to 30 minutes; of the kidney, after 50 to 100 minutes; and of the skin, after 6 to 12 hours. Although the shorter the time the organ is deprived of its blood supply the better, the cornea (角膜) can be removed for grafting(移植) at relative leisure, but every minute is of vital importance for a liver transplant.

B

When a kidney is removed from a living donor, it is not necessary to use elaborate preservation techniques. The operations on the donor and receiver are performed at the same time, and the receiver is prepared to receive the graft by the time that the donor organ is removed.

C

Cadaver(遗体) kidneys are removed as soon as possible after the donor's death, preferably within an hour. Cool solutions are put into the blood vessels of the kidney, which is then kept at 4℃ in a refrigerator or surrounded by ice in a vacuum bottle. At the same time, the receiver is prepared for operation.

D

Kidneys can be conserved(保存) in this simple way for 24 to 48 hours with little deterioration, and during this time they can be moved for long distances. For a kidney to be preserved from 48 to 72 hours, a complicated machine is required to provide artificial circulation. To keep a kidney undamaged for longer than 72 hours is difficult.

E

Blood cells, spermatozoa(精子) and certain other dissociated(游离的) tissue cells can be frozen to subzero temperatures and kept alive indefinitely.

F

Special preserving fluids will prevent cell destruction by ice crystals, but these fluids have damaging effects if introduced into whole organs such as the kidney.

Part Two

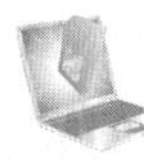

Questions 31—40

- Read the following passage.
- For each of the following sentences, decide whether it is **True (A)** or **False (B)**. If there is not enough information to answer **True (A)** or **False (B)**, choose **Not Given (C)**.
- Mark the corresponding letter on your **answer sheet.**

Prolonging Clinical Death

Modern scientists divide the process of dying into two phases—clinical or temporary death and biological death. Clinical death occurs when the organs, such as the heart or lungs, have ceased to function, but have not suffered permanent damage. The organism can still be revived. Biological death occurs when changes in the organism do permanent damage to cells and tissues. Death is then irreversible and final.

Scientists have been seeking a way to prolong the period of clinical death so that the organism can function again before biological death occurs. The best method developed so far involves cooling of the organism, combined with narcotic sleep(麻醉睡眠).

To illustrate how this works, scientists performed an experiment on a six-year-old female baboon(狒狒) called Keta. After narcotic, they surrounded her body with ice-bags and began checking her body temperature. When it had dropped to 28 degrees the scientists began draining blood from an artery. The monkey's blood pressure decreased and an hour later both the heart and respiration stopped; clinical death set in. Her temperature dropped to 22 degrees. At this point the scientists pumped blood into an artery in the direction of the heart and started artificial respiration. After two minutes the baboon's heart became active once more. After fifteen minutes, spontaneous respiration began, and after four hours Keta opened her eyes. Her behavior differed little from that of a healthy animal.

31. Modern scientists divide the process of dying into two phases—clinical death and biological death.

A. True **B.** False **C.** Not Given

32. One characteristic of biological death is temporary non-functioning of the heart.

A. True **B.** False **C.** Not Given

33. Scientists have been seeking a way to extend the period of clinical death.

A. True **B.** False **C.** Not Given

34. In the research, cooling the organism speeds up the damaging of body tissues.

A. True **B.** False **C.** Not Given

35. According to the passage, the young female baboon is the best experimental animal.

A. True **B.** False **C.** Not Given

36. According to the passage, Keta fell asleep with an anaesthetic.

A. True **B.** False **C.** Not Given

37. When Keta's temperature fell to 28 ℃, her blood pressure became higher and her heart stopped.

A. True **B.** False **C.** Not Given

38. When Keta's temperature fell to 22 ℃, scientists pumped blood into an artery and her respirations began immediately.

A. True **B.** False **C.** Not Given

39. The female baboon recovered its health after the experiment.

A. True **B.** False **C.** Not Given

40. One possible benefit from the experiment discussed in the passage is fewer deaths from heartattacks.

A. True **B.** False **C.** Not Given

Part Three

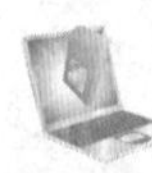

Questions 41—45

- Read the following passage.
- Choose the best answer **A**, **B** or **C**.
- Mark the corresponding letter on your **answer sheet**.

DNA

We all know that DNA has the ability to identify individuals but, because it is inherited, there are also regions of the DNA strand which can relate an individual to his or her family (immediate and extended), tribal group and even an entire population. Molecular Genealogy(宗谱学) can use this unique identification provided by the genetic markers to link people together into family trees. Pedigrees(家谱) based on such genetic markers can mean a breakthrough for family trees where information is incomplete or missing due to adoption, illegitimacy or lack of records. There are many communities and populations which have lost precious records due to tragic events such as the fire in the Irish courts during the Civil War in 1921 or American slaves for whom many records were never kept in the first place.

The main objective of the Molecular Genealogy Research Group is to build a database containing over 100, 000 DNA samples from individuals all over the world. These individuals will have provided a pedigree chart of at least four generations and a small blood sample. Once the database has enough samples to represent the world genetic make-up, it will eventually help in solving many issues, regarding genealogies that could not be done by relying only on traditional written records. Theoretically, any individual will someday be able to trace his or her family origins through this database.

In the meantime, as the database is being created, molecular genealogy can already verify possible or suspected relationships between individuals. "For example, if two men sharing the same last name believe that they are related, but no written record proves this relationship, we can verify this possibility by collecting a sample of DNA from both and looking for common markers in this case we can look primarily at the Y chromosome(染色体)," explain Ugo A. Perego, a member of the BYU Molecular Genealogy Research Group.

41. People in a large area may possess the same DNA thread because ________.

A. DNA is characteristic of a region

B. they are beyond doubt of common ancestry

C. DNA strand has the ability to identify individuals

42. Their possible research of family trees is based on the fact that ________.

A. genetics has achieved a breakthrough

B. genetics information contained in DNA can be revealed now

C. each individual carries a unique record of who he is related to others

43. The Molecular Genealogy Research Group is building a database for the purpose of ________.

A. offering assistance in working out genealogy-related problems

B. confirming the assumption that all individuals are of the same origin

C. providing a pedigree chart of at least four generations in the world

44. If two men suspected for some reason they have a common ancestor, ________.

A. we can decide according to their family tree

B. we can find the truth from their genetic makers

C. we can compare the differences in their Y chromosome

45. Which of the following CANNOT be inferred from the passage?

A. We are a waking, living, breathing record of our ancestors.

B. Many American slaves did not know who their ancestors were.

C. An adopted child generally lacks enough information to prove his identity.

Part Four >>>>>>

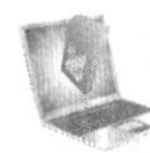

Questions 46—50

- Read the following procedures for using a hoist.
- Fill in each blank with the most appropriate procedure **A—F.** There is one extra procedure which you **DO NOT** need to use.
- Mark the corresponding letter on your **answer sheet.**

Procedures for Using a Hoist

Ⅰ. After operation, it's important to mobilize quickly in the Rehabilitation Unit. The Physiotherapists and nurses in the Rehab will help the patients to go for a short walk every day with a hoist. The steps are as follows:

Ⅱ. Firstly, **(46)** ________

Ⅲ. Next, bring the hoist to the patient and put up close.

Ⅳ. Then **(47)** ________

Ⅴ. Now, put the patient's feet into the slippers.

Ⅵ. Then **(48)** ________

Ⅶ. After that, ask the patient to hold on the bars with both hands.

Ⅷ. Next, **(49)** ________

Ⅸ. Finally, **(50)** ________

Ⅹ. Follow the steps and practice regularly; the patients will find it easy to use the equipment and make progress every day.

A. ask the patient to put his/her arms up and the nurse attaches the straps of the sling to the hoist.
B. the nurse explains what's going to happen and why it's important.
C. get the patient to go for a short walk.
D. take the patient to the wheelchair.
E. hoist the patient from sitting to stand position.
F. ask the patient to take a few steps.

Part Five >>>>>>

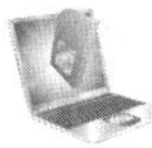

Questions 51—60

- Read the following passage.
- Choose the correct word for each blank from the list of words **A—L** given in the box below.
- Mark the corresponding letter on your **answer sheet.**

Losing Weight

About 70 million Americans are trying to lose weight. Some people go on (**51**) ________. This means they eat less of certain foods, especially (**52**) ________ and sugars. Other people exercise with special equipment, take diet pills, or even have (**53**) ________. Losing weight is hard work, and it can also cost a lot of money. So why do so many people in the United States want to lose weight?

Many people in the United States worry about not looking young and attractive. For many people, looking good also means being (**54**) ________. Other people worry about their (**55**) ________. Many doctors say being overweight is not healthy. But are Americans really fat?

Almost 30 million Americans weigh at least 20 percent more than their ideal weight. In fact, the United States is the most (**56**) ________ country in the world. "The (**57**) ________ fat of adult Americans weighs 2.3 trillion pounds," says University of Massachusetts anthropologist George Armelagos.

Losing weight is hard work, but most people want to find a (**58**) ________ and easy way to take (**59**) ________ fat. Bookstores sell lots of diet books. Each year, dozens of new books like these are written. Each one (**60**) ________ to get rid of fat.

A. surgery	**B.** diets	**C.** fast	**D.** overweight
E. on	**F.** health	**G.** stored	**H.** fats
I. promises	**J.** off	**K.** keep	**L.** thin

Part Six

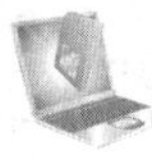

Questions 61

- Read the patient admission form below.
- Use the information to write a case report of **no less than 100 words.**
- Write the report on your **answer sheet.**

Patient Admission Form

Patient: Jasmine Miller — Age: 74

Gender: female — Date of Admission: Sep. 15, 2017

Chief Complaint:
- hypertension for one week

Signs and Symptoms:
- frequent urination
- increased thirst
- increased hunger
- dizziness
- feeling weak and fatigued

Diagnosis:
Diabetes

Nursing Instructions:
- inject insulin three times a day
- take medications for diabetes and hypertension
- have healthy diets, controlling sugar severely

医护英语水平考试（二级）

模拟训练（六）

Medical English Test System（METS）Level 2

I Listening

Part One

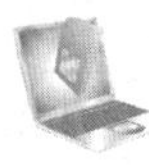

Questions 1—5

- You will hear five patients describing their problems. Decide what problem each patient has.
- Write the appropriate letter A—H in each box.
- Mark the corresponding letter on your **answer sheet**.
- You will hear each conversation twice.

Example:

0. Patient [E]

---

1. Patient 1 [ ]

2. Patient 2 [ ]

3. Patient 3 [ ]

4. Patient 4 [ ]

5. Patient 5 [ ]

A. Rash.

B. Pharyngitis.

C. Stroke.

D. Anemia.

E. Headache.

F. Stomachache.

G. Insomnia.

H. Heat-stroke.

Part Two

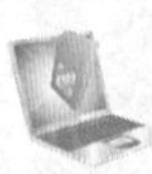

Questions 6—10

- You will hear a conversation between a patient and a doctor about diarrhea.
- For each of the following sentences, decide whether it is **True (A)** or **False (B)**. Put a tick (√) in the relevant box.
- Mark the corresponding letter on your **answer sheet**.

- You will hear the conversation twice.

Example:

0. The patient went to hospital because of headache.

A. True ☐
B. False ☑

---

6. Mr. Johnson has been in the toilets for over 10 times since last night.

A. True ☐
B. False ☐

7. There is always some mucus in Mr. Johnson's stool.

A. True ☐
B. False ☐

8. Mr. Johnson has been vomiting for hours.

A. True ☐
B. False ☐

9. Mr. Johnson needs a stool test.

A. True ☐
B. False ☐

10. The doctor will give Mr. Johnson intravenous injection to prevent dehydration.

A. True ☐
B. False ☐

Part Three

Questions 11—15

- You will hear a conversation between a patient and a doctor about heartburn.
- For each of the following questions or unfinished sentences, choose the correct answer **A**, **B** or **C**. Put a tick (√) in the relevant box.
- Mark the corresponding letter on your **answer sheet**.
- You will hear the conversation twice.

---

11. What can we know about heartburn from the dialogue?

A. The stomach acid goes up into the mouth. ☐
B. It only happens before meals. ☐

	C. It's a problem with heart.	☐
12. When did the patient's problem get worse?	**A.** One month ago.	☐
	B. Two weeks ago.	☐
	C. Eighteen months ago.	☐
13. When did the patient get heartburn?	**A.** Shortly before meals.	☐
	B. Shortly after meals.	☐
	C. Long after meals.	☐
14. How does the patient think about heartburn?	**A.** It is unpleasant.	☐
	B. It is aching.	☐
	C. It is chronic.	☐
15. Why did the nurse tell the patient her own problem?	**A.** To advise him to over-eat.	☐
	B. To seek his sympathy.	☐
	C. To reassure his emotions.	☐

Part Four >>>>>>

Questions 16—20

- You will hear a conversation between a doctor and a patient about the treatment of fracture.
- Fill in the blanks.
- Write the answers on your **answer sheet.**
- You will hear the conversation twice.

SURNAME Simon		
AGE 39	SEX M	**MARITAL STATUS** M

OCCUPATION Cook
What Happened? The patient was (**16**) ________ to the ground by a car. The patient's left arm and elbow were grazed and had a pain in his (**17**) ________.
Examination A(n) (**18**) ________ examination.
Diagnosis A hairline (**19**) ________.
Treatment No need for plaster. Some (**20**) ________ medicine, oral medicine and a tube of ointment.
POINTS TO NOTE Take two or three weeks off work, and rest in bed as much as possible.

Ⅱ Reading and Writing

Part One

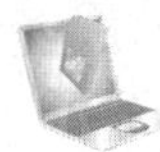

Questions 21—30

- Read the descriptions of obesity.
- Decide which part (**A**—**F**) mentions this (**21**—**30**). Some parts may be chosen more than once. Sentence **0** is an example.
- For each of the following questions, choose the correct answer **A**—**F**. Write the answer in the relevant box.
- Mark the corresponding letter on your **answer sheet**.

Which part(s) mention(s) that

- the number of overweight children has increased? | **0** | A |
- food marketing and poor policymaking result in the world's obesity problem? | **21** | |

- obesity means there are large amounts of fat in your body? **22** ___
- healthy food is so expensive that poor people can't afford? **23** ___
- the growth of childhood obesity has slowed in countries where wages are higher? **24** ___
- you could hardly see a lot of obese children a few decades ago? **25** ___
- 130 million people were examined in this research? **26** ___
- some cancers result from obesity? **27** ___
- east Asia is one of the Middle Income Countries areas? **28** ___
- children's school performance is influenced by obesity? **29** ___
- the Body Mass Index measurements are related to height and weight? **30** ___

A

A new study provides evidence of a sharp increase in the number of obese and overweight children and young adults worldwide in just 40 years. The study was a project of researchers at Imperial College London and the World Health Organization (WHO). Obesity is a condition in which the body stores large, unhealthy amounts of fat. Obese individuals are considered overweight.

B

The researchers studied obesity rates among children and young people, between 5 and 19 years of age. They found that rates in this group increased from 11 million in 1975 to 124 million in 2016. This was one of the biggest epidemiological studies ever done. The researchers examined height and weight data for about 130 million people. They used this information to get the Body Mass Index measurements of the subjects.

C

The most striking changes have taken place in Middle Income Countries in areas such as East Asia, the Middle East and North Africa, and Latin America. The WHO defines Middle Income Countries as places where a person normally earns between $1,045 and $12,736 every year.

D

Majid Ezzati, a professor at Imperial College London, was the chief writer of a report on the study. He was surprised by the speed of change. "So places that a few decades ago, there may have been very little obesity and a fair amount of underweight children, suddenly are having bordering epidemics." In countries where wages are higher, the growth of childhood obesity has slowed, but remains high. The United States had the highest obesity rates for this income group. Researchers say the world's obesity problem is a result of food marketing and poor policymaking in many areas.

E

Ezzati notes that, in general, young people are not to blame. "Rather than sort of being an individual's choice, it's hard environments that people choose their foods in—healthy foods being priced out of reach, and especially out of reach of poor, and unhealthy foods being marketed aggressively, together with perhaps not having a safe playing area for children, that are leading to weight gain."

F

Being overweight can cause many diseases later in life, including heart disease, stroke, diabetes and some cancers. Ezzati says obesity also has a big effect on children, with some evidence suggesting it can affect their educational performance.

Part Two >>>>>>

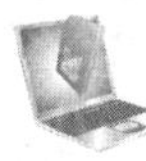

Questions 31—40

- Read the following passage.
- For each of the following sentences, decide whether it is **True** (**A**) or **False** (**B**). If there is not enough information to answer **True** (**A**) or **False** (**B**), choose **Not Given** (**C**).
- Mark the corresponding letter on your **answer sheet**.

Exercises to Help "Tech Neck"

When we do the same movements with our bodies over and over again, we overuse some muscles. And that overuse can lead to strain and injury. Sometimes those problems can come from doing sports. But exercise professionals say they are now seeing another cause for muscle problems: hand-held technology devices.

Staring down at your phone or tablet for long periods of time puts great tension on your neck and spine. Many people who use tech devices also hunch their shoulders forward. Experts say this posture puts strain on the entire upper body. Muscle strain linked to hand-held technology has become such a common condition that it now has a name: tech neck.

Kimberly Fielding, an exercise teacher in New York City, explains that constantly looking down at our devices creates an unnatural curve in our spine. This can cause nerve pain and other problems. "A lot of the curves of the neck can change, so instead of the cervical spine going inward, the curve can be a little bit different and it causes nerve pain and herniation(s) and different muscle tension headaches—different things that really can reduce quality of life."

Common symptoms of tech neck are neck pain, loss of feeling in your hands and fingers, headaches—both mild and severe—and poor posture. In the worst cases of tech neck, you can lose the strength in your hands and fingers. Fielding noticed that many of her clients were coming to her for help with this "forward head posture". So, she created a class to directly address the problem of tech neck. The class uses different exercises to release tension in the upper body and strengthen back and neck muscles. The class also works on breathing and posture.

However, you don't need to take a class like Fielding's. You can take simple steps to improve tech neck. Take breaks from using your technology. Stand up and stretch your legs often. Also, give your eyes a break by closing them throughout the day. Move your eyes to the screen, not your neck, head or shoulders. Do neck exercises.

And if your tech neck symptoms get worse, see a health care professional.

31. Overuse of some muscles can result in strain and injury.
A. True **B.** False **C.** Not Given

32. Those who use tech devices often shrug their shoulders.
A. True **B.** False **C.** Not Given

33. Abnormal curve in our spine can cause nerve pain and other problems.
A. True **B.** False **C.** Not Given

34. Watching too much TV is harmful to the neck.
A. True **B.** False **C.** Not Given

35. Nerve pain and tension headaches can reduce quality of life.
A. True **B.** False **C.** Not Given

36. One of the common symptoms of tech neck is headache.
A. True **B.** False **C.** Not Given

37. You may lose your fingers if your tech neck gets worse.
A. True **B.** False **C.** Not Given

38. Fielding's class helped her clients with tech neck problems.
A. True **B.** False **C.** Not Given

39. Holding your phone at eye level can release tension in the upper body.
A. True **B.** False **C.** Not Given

40. To improve your tech neck, you can move your head or neck to the screen.
A. True **B.** False **C.** Not Given

Part Three

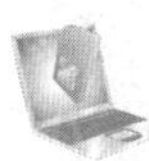

Questions 41—45

- Read the following passage.
- Choose the best answer **A**, **B** or **C**.
- Mark the corresponding letter on your **answer sheet**.

Your Stomach and Brain Are Connected

A new study provides more evidence that there is a deep connection between our gut and our brains. The findings suggest that **probiotics**—so-called "good" bacteria that aid in digestion—may also help to lessen symptoms of depression.

There are about 300 to 500 bacterial species that live in the human gut. Many help with digestion and keep the gastrointestinal system working right.

Scientists say these probiotics play a part in neural activity that controls digestion. In addition, there is also new evidence that shows probiotics can also affect a person's mental state, or mood.

Premysl Bercik is a researcher at Ontario Canada's McMaster University. Bercik is interested in the connection between the gut and the brain through the millions of bacteria that live in the gastrointestinal tract. Bercik notes that between 40 and 90 percent of people with irritable bowel syndrome, or IBS, also suffer from symptoms of anxiety and depression.

Doctors do not yet know what causes IBS. It causes stomach pains and can interfere with the body's waste removal process. The difficulty and discomfort of the condition alone might cause depression. However, research led by Bercik suggests that the presence or lack of gut bacteria may affect a person's mood.

"What we found was that the patients who were treated with this probiotic bacterium improved their gut's symptoms, but also surprisingly decreased their depression scores. That means their mood improved. And this was associated also with changes in the brain imaging."

Bercik says larger studies are needed to confirm the findings. The researchers will publish their findings in the journal *Gastroenterology*.

41. The underlined word **probiotics** in Paragraph 1 means ________.

A. a kind of beneficial microbes

B. a kind of harmful germs

C. a kind of medicine

42. Which of the following is NOT TRUE about probiotics?

A. Probiotics may help with digestion.
B. Probiotics can help cure depression.
C. Probiotics can be found in the human gut.

43. New evidence shows that ________.
A. probiotics have an effect on one's mood
B. probiotics play a role in bowel movement
C. there are many types of probiotics in the human gut

44. Which of the following is NOT the symptom of IBS?
A. Anxiety. **B.** Stomach pain. **C.** Difficulty urinating.

45. Which of the following statements is TRUE according to the passage?
A. Over half of Canadian people suffer from irritable bowel syndrome.
B. Studies found that patients with mental illness could be treated with probiotics.
C. Patients treated with probiotics improved their mood as well as their gut's symptoms.

Part Four >>>>>>

Questions 46—50

- Read the following procedures for an MRI scan.
- Fill in each blank with the most appropriate procedure **A—F.** There is one extra procedure which you **DO NOT** need to use.
- Mark the corresponding letter on your **answer sheet.**

How Do You Prepare for an MRI Scan?

Ⅰ. All metallic objects on the body are removed prior to obtaining an MRI scan. Occasionally, you will be given a sedative medication to decrease anxiety and relax yourself during the MRI scan.

Ⅱ. **(46)** ________ Depending on the part of your body being scanned, you'll be moved into the scanner either head first or feet first.

Ⅲ. The MRI scanner is operated by a radiographer, who is trained in carrying out imaging investigations. **(47)** ________

Ⅳ. **(48)** ________

Ⅴ. At certain times during the scan, the scanner will make loud tapping noises. This is the electric current in the scanner coils being turned on and off. **(49)** ________

Ⅵ. **(50)** ________ The scan lasts 15 to 90 minutes, depending on the size of the area being scanned and how many images are taken.

A. You'll be given earplugs or headphones to wear.
B. You'll be able to talk to the radiographer through an intercom and they'll be able to see you on a television monitor throughout the scan.
C. The radiographer controls the scanner using a computer, which is in a different room, to keep it away from the magnetic field generated by the scanner.
D. It's very important to keep as still as possible during your MRI scan.
E. During an MRI scan, you lie on a flat bed that's moved into the scanner.
F. Interaction with the MRI technologist is maintained throughout the test.

Part Five

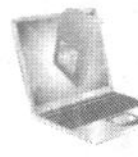

Questions 51—60

- Read the following passage.
- Choose the correct word for each blank from the list of words **A—L** given in the box below.
- Mark the corresponding letter on your **answer sheet**.

Vitamin D Deficiency

Vitamin D deficiency means that you are not getting enough vitamin D to stay healthy.

Vitamin D helps your body (**51**) ________ calcium. Calcium is one of the main building blocks of bone. Vitamin D also has a (**52**) ________ in your nervous, muscle, and immune systems. You can get vitamin D in three ways: through your skin, from your diet, and from (**53**) ________. Your body forms vitamin D naturally after (**54**) ________ to sunlight. But too much sun exposure can lead to skin aging and skin cancer, so many people try to get their vitamin D from other sources.

You can become deficient in vitamin D for different reasons: You don't get enough vitamin D in your diet; You don't get enough exposure to sunlight.

Vitamin D deficiency can lead to a loss of bone (**55**) ________, which can (**56**) ________ to osteoporosis and fractures. Severe vitamin D deficiency can also lead to other diseases. In children, it can cause rickets. Rickets is a rare disease that causes the bones to become soft and (**57**) ________. African American infants and children are at higher risk of getting rickets. In adults, severe vitamin D deficiency leads to osteomalacia. Osteomalacia causes (**58**) ________ bones, bone pain, and muscle weakness.

Researchers are studying vitamin D for its (**59**) ________ connections to several medical conditions, including diabetes, high blood pressure, cancer, and autoimmune conditions such as multiple sclerosis. They need to do more research before they can understand the (**60**) ________ of vitamin D on these conditions.

A. density	**B**. weak	**C**. exposure	**D**. bend
E. possible	**F**. absorb	**G**. usage	**H**. role
I. cause	**J**. effects	**K**. supplements	**L**. contribute

Part Six >>>>>>

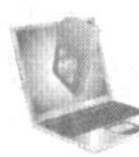

Questions 61

- Read the patient admission form below.
- Use the information to write a case report of **no less than 100 words.**
- Write the report on your **answer sheet.**

Patient Admission Form

Patient: John Brown
Age: 56
Gender: male
Date of Admission: July 7, 2017

Chief complaint:
- cough
- chest pain
- shortness of breath

Signs and symptoms:
- T:37.8 ℃
- severe cough
- difficulty breathing
- productive yellow and greenish sputum

Diagnosis:
chronic bronchitis

Nursing instructions:
- drink much water and have a good rest
- do not have spicy food
- do not smoke or drink alcohol
- use some cough medicine and antibiotics if necessary

医护英语水平考试（二级）

模拟训练（七）

Medical English Test System（METS）Level 2

Ⅰ Listening

Part One

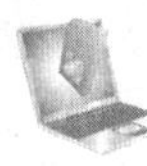

Questions 1—5

- You will hear patients describing their pains. Decide what kind of pain each patient has.
- Write the appropriate letter **A**—**H** in each box.
- Mark the corresponding letter on your **answer sheet.**
- You will hear each conversation twice.

Example:

0. Health **F**

---

1. Adams ☐

2. Johns ☐

3. Green ☐

4. Wilson ☐

5. Dan ☐

A. Dull pain.

B. Stinging pain.

C. Burning pain.

D. Stabbing pain.

E. Tingling pain.

F. Numbness.

G. Throbbing pain.

H. Sharp pain.

Part Two

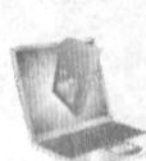

Questions 6—10

- You will hear a conversation between a patient and a doctor about health problem.
- For each of the following sentences, decide whether it is **True (A)** or **False (B)**. Put a tick (√) in the relevant box.

- Mark the corresponding letter on your **answer sheet**.
- You will hear the conversation twice.

Example:

0. The patient works at a university.	**A.** True	✓
	B. False	☐

6. The patient has got a very serious lump of fibrosis tissue.	**A.** True	☐
	B. False	☐
7. The lump won't disappear by itself.	**A.** True	☐
	B. False	☐
8. It is not a cancer but a benign tumor.	**A.** True	☐
	B. False	☐
9. The patient felt at ease when she was told to be hospitalized for the operation.	**A.** True	☐
	B. False	☐
10. The patient finally agreed to have the operation.	**A.** True	☐
	B. False	☐

Part Three

Questions 11—15

- You will hear a conversation between a patient and a doctor about his disease.
- For each of the following questions or unfinished sentences, choose the correct answer **A**, **B** or **C**. Put a tick (✓) in the relevant box.
- Mark the corresponding letter on your **answer sheet**.
- You will hear the conversation twice.

11. What disease does Mr. Jones have?	**A.** Obesity.	☐
	B. Diabetes.	☐
	C. Stroke.	☐

12. What does the doctor advise Mr. Jones to give up?
A. Smoking. ☐
B. Eating desserts. ☐
C. Drinking juice. ☐

13. What may help move Mr. Jones' attention away from alcohol and desserts?
A. Listening to music. ☐
B. Reading novels. ☐
C. Both A and B. ☐

14. What is Mr. Jones' another problem?
A. He can't see well. ☐
B. He can't hear clearly. ☐
C. He is unable to sleep. ☐

15. What needs to be done before the eye operation?
A. Controlling the blood pressure. ☐
B. Controlling the weight. ☐
C. Controlling the blood glucose. ☐

Part Four

Questions 16—20

- You will hear a conversation between a nurse and a patient about her vital signs.
- Fill in the blanks.
- Write the answers on your **answer sheet**.
- You will hear the conversation twice.

Full Name Jenny Thompson
Present Complaint The patient (**16**) ________ so much that she felt she was going to pass out.
Examination The nurse would insert the probe into the patient's mouth to measure her (**17**) ________. The nurse would take the patient's (**18**) ________ by the radial site. The nurse would take the patient's (**19**) ________ saturation since she was a little short of breath.

Results
T: 39 ℃
P: 110 bpm
RR: 35 bpm, (**20**) ________ but shallow and quick.
BP: 120/80 mmHg

Ⅱ Reading and Writing

Part One

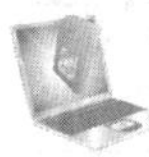

Questions 21—30

- Read the descriptions of ways to lubricate dry eyes.
- Decide which part (**A**—**F**) mentions this (**21**—**30**). Some parts may be chosen more than once. Sentence **0** is an example.
- For each of the following questions, choose the correct answer **A**—**F**. Write the answer in the relevant box.
- Mark the corresponding letter on your **answer sheet**.

Which part(s) mention(s)

- preservative free solutions? **0** E
- moisture generated by humidifier? **21** ____
- dry eyes caused by reading or watching TV? **22** ____
- dry eyes caused by excessive air movement? **23** ____
- warm compresses in dealing with inflammation of the eyelids? **24** ____
- the difference between lubricating eye ointments and eyedrops? **25** ____
- use of artificial tears and lubricating eyedrops? **26** ____
- drawing the oil out of the glands by massaging? **27** ____
- decreasing the speed of ceiling fans to avoid dry eyes? **28** ____
- decrease of humidity caused by air conditioners? **29** ____
- the proper time to use eye oinments? **30** ____

A

If you notice your eyes are dry mainly while reading or watching TV, taking frequent breaks to allow the eyes to rest and become moist may be helpful.

B

Excessive air movement dries out your eyes. Avoid this by decreasing the speed of ceiling fans and/or oscillating fans.

C

A humidifier puts more moisture in the air. With more moisture in the air, tears evaporate more slowly, keeping your eyes more comfortable. Also, both furnaces and air conditioners decrease humidity in the air.

D

Warm compresses and eyelid scrubs with baby shampoo help provide a thicker, more stable layer of lubricant. This is especially helpful if you have inflammation of the eyelids or problems with the glands in your eyelid that make the lubricant. The heat warms up the oil in the glands, making it flow more easily; the massaging action helps draw the oil out of the glands. The cleansing action decreases the number of bacteria that break down the oil.

E

Artificial tears and lubricating eyedrops and gels (available over the counter) help provide more moisture and lubrication for the surface of your eye. They are typically used about four times a day, but can be used as often as needed. Preservative free solutions are recommended if you wish to use tears more than six times a day.

F

Lubricating eye ointments are much thicker than eyedrops and gels. Because ointments are so thick, they last much longer than eyedrops and gels. However, because of their thickness, ointments may blur your vision if used during the day. Therefore, they are typically used to lubricate the eyes overnight while you sleep.

Part Two >>>>>>

Questions 31—40

- Read the following passage.
- For each of the following sentences, decide whether it is **True (A)** or **False (B)**. If there is not enough information to answer **True (A)** or **False (B)**, choose **Not Given (C)**.
- Mark the corresponding letter on your **answer sheet.**

Your Doctor and Your Headache

Many headache sufferers do not consult a doctor. A recent study showed that 50% of migraine sufferers had not sought medical advice and had not been diagnosed with migraine. As a result, they were not being treated for migraine.

Many people are disabled by headache. They may receive sympathy from relatives, friends and colleagues but this does not ease the pain. They may take and be prescribed medication that was not very effective.

It is important that you consult your doctor to diagnose your headache. Any severe or constant headache that begins suddenly and is accompanied by weakness, dizziness, numbness or other strange physical sensations should be reported to a doctor immediately.

Your doctor should be consulted if you have frequent debilitating(衰弱的) headaches or take an excessive number of pain relievers. The appointment should be made to specifically discuss the headache.

The role of your doctor is to accurately diagnose your headache and then to work with you to help minimize the effect it has on you and your lifestyle. Recommending medication is a part of this process. As with any medical problem, it is important to have enough specialized knowledge about headache or may not take headache seriously. Make sure your doctor is aware of the disability caused by headache to your quality of life and how it affects your partner, children, employer, work colleagues and friends.

Headache management is a great challenge. A number of treatment options, preparations and methods of administration may have to be tried to discover what works best for each headache sufferer. The role of the doctor is vital in this process. Once your headache is correctly diagnosed, your headache management plan can be developed. The plan should be evaluated and updated regularly.

Patient-doctor communication is vital for the best outcome. Effective communication on both sides can result in a trial-and-error process that leads to effective treatment that will minimize the pain and disability associated with headache.

31. Many headache sufferers do not seek medical advice.

A. True **B.** False **C.** Not Given

32. Because of misdiagnoses, 50% of migraine sufferers were not treated for migraine.

A. True **B.** False **C.** Not Given

33. Sympathy from relatives and friends can ease the pain.

A. True **B.** False **C.** Not Given

34. Severe headache with dizziness should be reported to a doctor immediately.

A. True **B.** False **C.** Not Given

35. You should consult your doctor before stopping the use of pain relievers.

A. True **B**. False **C**. Not Given

36. Doctors will give you advice on the proper use of medication.

A. True **B**. False **C**. Not Given

37. You should tell your doctor how headache affects your life and your friends.

A. True **B**. False **C**. Not Given

38. Due to many treatment options, headache management is not difficult.

A. True **B**. False **C**. Not Given

39. Doctors are very important in discovering the best treatment for your headache.

A. True **B**. False **C**. Not Given

40. Effective patient-doctor communication can lead to effective treatment.

A. True **B**. False **C**. Not Given

Part Three

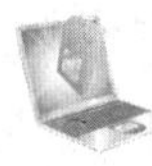

Questions 41—45

- Read the following passage.
- Choose the best answer **A**, **B** or **C**.
- Mark the corresponding letter on your **answer sheet**.

Older People Are Under Threat from Loneliness

Feeling isolated is not only soul destroying, it's also a risk factor for early death. Macbeth may have spoken of "that which should accompany old age, such as honor, love, obedience, troops of friends", but here and now old people are more likely to be bitterly lonely, according to a paper by Marcus Rand of *The Campaign to End Loneliness*. It seems that about one in ten of people over 65 feel chronically lonely all or most of the time.

A lot of this is due to things we think of as benefits: easy transport so people have no need to go on living where they grew up and maybe elders in the family still live; and the ability to make arrangements online, using digital skills which older people may not have.

Interestingly, organizations concerned with older people regard loneliness as a health problem as well as a social one. A lack of social connections is "a risk factor for early death", which can be compared to smoking 15 cigarettes a day and is worse for the elderly than obesity and physical inactivity, according to *The Campaign to End Loneliness* website.

Janet Morrison of *Independent Age* deplores the level of **stigma** and negative attitudes towards loneliness, and says we need to help local authorities and the public accept that "there's nothing wrong with admitting to being lonely, and things can be done to help reduce it"—though I don't think she would approve of the old suggestion of standing in a busy market with a lasso.

Morrison says we must help local authorities realize that being lonely is not normal or necessary. The irony of all this is that those who may be old and lonely now are the ones who may well have thought in 1960s that youth and only youth was worth living or thinking about. Perhaps this sort of punishment comes to us all.

41. How many people over 65 feel chronically lonely all or most of the time?

A. One per cent.

B. Ten per cent.

C. Twenty per cent.

42. Which of the following may NOT cause loneliness of old people?

A. Easy access to transport means.

B. Growing up with older generations.

C. The ability to manage everything via Internet.

43. Why dose the author compare a lack of social connections to heavy smoking?

A. Because it may cause early death.

B. Because it may cause obesity.

C. Because it may cause physical inactivity.

44. What dose the word "stigma" in Paragraph 4 refer to?

A. Something to be in favor of.

B. Something to be proud of.

C. Something to be ashamed of.

45. Which of the following is Morrison's view?

A. Old people are likely to be bitterly lonely now.

B. Things can be done to help reduce loneliness.

C. Only youth is worth living or thinking about.

Part Four

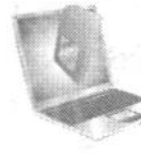

Questions 46—50

- Read the following procedures for using an Automated External Defibrillator (AED)(自动体外除颤器).
- Fill in each blank with the most appropriate procedure **A—F.** There is one extra procedure which you **DO NOT** need to use.
- Mark the corresponding letter on your **answer sheet.**

How to Use an Automated External Defibrillator (AED)

AEDs are user-friendly devices that untrained bystanders can use to save the life of someone having sudden cardiac arrest.

Ⅰ. If you see a person suddenly collapse and pass out, or already unconscious, call 120 and check the person's breathing and pulse. If breathing and pulse are absent or irregular, prepare to use the AED as soon as possible.

Ⅱ. (**46**) ________

Ⅲ. Turn on the AED's power. The device will give you step-by-step instructions. You'll hear voice prompts and see prompts on a screen.

Ⅳ. Expose the person's chest. Remove metal necklaces and underwire bras. The metal may conduct electricity and cause burns. You can cut the center of the bra and pull it away from the skin.

Ⅴ. AEDs have sticky pads with sensors called electrodes. Place one pad on the right center of the person's chest above the nipple. (**47**) ________

Ⅵ. (**48**) ________ Stay clear while the machine checks the person's heart rhythm.

Ⅶ. If a shock is needed, the AED will let you know when to deliver it. Stand clear of the person and make sure others are clear before you push the AED's "shock" button.

Ⅷ. (**49**) ________

Ⅸ. If the person starts moving, coughing, or breathing regularly, place the person in a recovery position and keep him or her as still as possible.

Ⅹ. (**50**) ________

A. Do not remove the pads or disconnect them from the defibrillator until emergency medical personnel arrive.

B. Before using an AED, move the person to a dry area, and stay away from wetness when delivering shocks (water conducts electricity).

C. Make sure no one is touching the person, and then press the AED's "analyze" button.

D. Place the electrode pad over an implanted device such as an implanted pacemaker or ICD.

E. Remember, once the AED delivers a shock, immediately deliver 5 cycles of CPR (approximately 2 minutes' compressions).

F. Place the other pad slightly below the other nipple and to the left of the ribcage.

Part Five

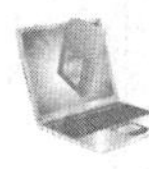

Questions 51—60

- Read the following passage.
- Choose the correct word for each blank from the list of words **A**—**L** given in the box below.
- Mark the corresponding letter on your **answer sheet**.

Alzheimer's Disease

Alzheimer's disease (AD) is a chronic neurodegenerative disease that usually starts slowly and worsens over time. The most common early symptom is difficulty in remembering recent events—short-term memory (**51**) ________. As the disease advances, symptoms can include problems with language, disorientation (including easily getting lost), mood swings, loss of (**52**) ________, not managing self-care, and behavioural issues. As a person's condition declines, they often withdraw from family and society. Gradually, bodily functions are lost, ultimately leading to death. Although the speed of (**53**) ________ can vary, the average life expectancy following diagnosis is three to nine years.

The cause of Alzheimer's disease is poorly understood. About 70% of the risk is believed to be (**54**) ________ with many genes usually involved. Other risk factors include a history of head injuries, depression, or hypertension. A probable diagnosis is (**55**) ________ on the history of the illness and cognitive testing with medical imaging and blood tests to rule out other possible causes. Initial symptoms are often mistaken for normal (**56**) ________. Examination of brain tissue is needed for a definite diagnosis. Mental and physical exercise, and avoiding obesity may (**57**) ________ the risk of AD; however, evidence to support these recommendations is not strong. There are no medications or supplements that decrease risk.

No treatments stop or (**58**) ________ its progression, though some may temporarily improve symptoms. Affected people increasingly rely on others for assistance, often placing a burden on the caregiver; the pressures can include social, psychological, physical and (**59**) ________ elements. Exercise programs may be (**60**) ________ with respect to activities of daily living and can potentially improve outcomes.

A. reverse	**B.** motivation	**C.** based	**D.** loss
E. beneficial	**F.** genetic	**G.** economic	**H.** infectious
I. decrease	**J.** ageing	**K.** progression	**L.** harmful

Part Six >>>>>>

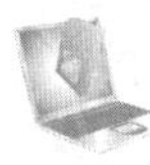

Questions 61

- Read the patient discharge summary below.
- Use the information to write a case report of **no less than 100 words.**
- Write the report on your **answer sheet.**

Discharge Summary
Patient: Martin Downes **Age:** 43 **Gender:** male **Date of Discharge:** 01/05/2017 **Date of Admission:** 24/04/2017
Reason for Admission: • 4 days of frequency & urgency of urine • 20 days of repeated cough and fever
PE on Admission: • Harsh respiratory sound • Heart murmurs
Diagnosis on Admission: • Interstitial pneumonia • UTI (urinary tract infection) • Secondary fungus infection
Medication and Treatment: • Anti-infection, anti-virus, eliminating phlegm • Improving immunity • Anti-fungus infection
Present Condition: In good condition
Needs: • Drink water. • Take enough rest.

听力文本、参考答案及解析

医护英语水平考试(二级)

模拟训练(一)

听力文本

This is METS-2 listening test. There are four parts in the test, Parts One, Two, Three, and Four. You will hear each part twice. Now, look at the instructions for Part One.
You will hear five patients describing their problems. Decide what problem each patient has. Write the appropriate letter A-H in each box. Mark the corresponding letter on your answer sheet. You will hear each conversation twice.

Here is an example:

Nurse (Woman): Good morning. What seems to be your problem?
Patient (Man): I have a pain in my stomach.
Nurse (Woman): Did you vomit?
Patient (Man): No, I didn't.
The answer is stomachache, so write letter F in the box. Now we are ready to start.

Conversation 1

Nurse (Woman): Good morning. What seems to be the trouble?
Patient (Man): I cannot sleep well these days. My head hurts.
Nurse (Woman): How long have you had this problem?
Patient (Man): About one week.

Conversation 2

Nurse (Woman): What's troubling you, Mr. Black?
Patient (Man): I have a sore throat.
Nurse (Woman): Let me take a look at your throat. Open your mouth and say "ah".
Patient (Man): Ah.
Nurse (Woman): Look, your throat is inflamed. You have the symptoms of flu.

Conversation 3

Nurse (Woman): You don't look well, Jack. What happened?
Patient (Man): Well, I fell off my bike and my left leg was wounded.
Nurse (Woman): Let me have a look. Oh, there is a cut and it's bleeding. Does it hurt when I press here?
Patient (Man): No, there is no pain.
Nurse (Woman): Don't worry. Let's sterilize it first.

Conversation 4

Nurse (Woman): What's wrong with you, Mr. Green?
Patient (Man): The joints in my right arm ache.
Nurse (Woman): How long have you been like this?
Patient (Man): For more than one year. At first I didn't care because I ride motorcycle too much, but now my whole right arm is not as flexible as it used to be.

Conversation 5

Nurse (Woman): You look pale, Mr. White. What's your problem?
Patient (Man): I cough severely and have a pain in the chest. My temperature reached 38 degrees centigrade this morning.
Nurse (Woman): Do you have difficulty in breathing?
Patient (Man): Yes, I can't breathe easily.
Nurse (Woman): How long have you been like this?
Patient (Man): For about three days.

This is the end of Part One. Now look at Part Two. You will hear a conversation between a patient and a nurse about health problem. For each of the following sentences, decide whether it is True (A) or False (B). Put a tick (√) in the relevant box. Mark the corresponding letter on your answer sheet. You will hear the conversation twice.

Nurse (Woman): Good evening, Mr. Green! What's wrong with you?
Patient (Man): Good evening, Nurse. I'm not feeling well today. I have a pain in my abdomen.
Nurse (Woman): How long have you had it?
Patient (Man): It started in the morning. At the beginning I had a stomachache.
Nurse (Woman): How long did it last?
Patient (Man): About 3 hours, but this afternoon it moved to the lower right part of the abdomen for 5 hours.
Nurse (Woman): Have you had any vomiting?

Patient (Man): I have only nausea.
Nurse (Woman): Have you had any diarrhea?
Patient (Man): No.
Nurse (Woman): Any fever?
Patient (Man): I don't know.
Nurse (Woman): Let me take your temperature. All right, you have a slight fever. Please lie down on the bed; loosen your belt, please. Let the doctor examine your abdomen.
Patient (Man): Thank you.
Nurse (Woman): Don't be nervous and try to relax.
Patient (Man): All right.
Nurse (Woman): The result of your blood test tells us that your white blood cell count is 18,000. The doctor said that you had acute appendicitis.
Patient (Man): Oh, I am scared.
Nurse (Woman): Don't be afraid, you will recover. The doctor said that you have to have an operation. So, please sign your name on the consent form to say that you agree to the operation on you.
Patient (Man): No problem.
Nurse (Woman): Thanks for your cooperation.

This is the end of Part Two. Now look at Part Three. You will hear a conversation between a patient and a doctor about Traditional Chinese Medicine (TCM). For each of the following questions or unfinished sentences, choose the correct answer A, B or C. Put a tick (√) in the relevant box. Mark the corresponding letter on your answer sheet. You will hear the conversation twice.

Doctor (Woman): Hello, Mr. Smith. How are you feeling today?
Patient (Man): Much better, thank you, Dr. Brown! I can sit straight today. The acupuncture is really great.
Doctor (Woman): Yes, traditional Chinese medicine, or TCM, has a history of more than 5,000 years. TCM has a complete theory about the occurrence, development and treatment of diseases. Acupuncture is only one of the most effective ways to treat some diseases such as yours.
Patient (Man): Would you please tell me more about TCM?
Doctor (Woman): OK. According to the TCM theory, the occurrence of diseases is the incoordination between Yin and Yang and the treatment of diseases is the reestablishment of the balance between them.
Patient (Man): Oh, what are Yin and Yang?
Doctor (Woman): They are the two concepts from ancient Chinese philosophy and they represent the two contradictories in everything. In the TCM theory, Yin and Yang are

used to explain physiological and pathological phenomena of the body. They are also the principles of diagnosing and treating diseases.

Patient (Man): That's really fantastic.

Doctor (Woman): To tell the truth, according to statistics, traditional Chinese medicine is better for the treatment of diseases of viral infection, immune system and nervous system without causing any side effects compared with Western medicine.

Patient (Man): Thank you very much, Doctor. I've got better understanding of TCM now.

This is the end of Part Three. Now look at Part Four. You will hear a conversation between a doctor and a patient about the treatment of wound. Fill in the blanks. Write the answers on your answer sheet. You will hear the conversation twice.

Doctor (Woman): Good morning. What's your surname?

Patient (Man): It's Tweedie.

Doctor (Woman): That's T-W-E-E-D-I-E. Is that right?

Patient (Man): Yes.

Doctor (Woman): Well, what's the trouble, Mr. Tweedie?

Patient (Man): I have a wound in my head here. It really hurts.

Doctor (Woman): How did it happen?

Patient (Man): I tripped and fell, banging my head quite hard. My wife wrapped a bandage around it to stop the bleeding.

Doctor (Woman): Did you lose a lot of blood?

Patient (Man): Not too much.

Doctor (Woman): Were you unconscious then?

Patient (Man): No, I wasn't.

Doctor (Woman): The wound is rather large, so I'll stitch it up.

Patient (Man): Will it hurt?

Doctor (Woman): Oh, no. It won't be painful. We'll give you a local anesthesia. By the way, have you had an anti-tetanus injection lately?

Patient (Man): I think the only one I have had was about 5 years ago.

Doctor (Woman): Well, I think you'd better have another one.

Patient (Man): OK.

Doctor (Woman): Come again in 3 days and we'll re-examine the wound.

Patient (Man): All right. Thank you very much.

This is the end of Part Four. You now have five minutes to write your answers on the answer sheet. You have one more minute. This is the end of the listening test.

参考答案及解析

Ⅰ Listening

Part One

1. G　本题中病人自述因头痛而失眠，故选 G。

2. H　本题病人咽喉痛，通过观察，属于流感(flu)症状，故选 H。

3. C　病人自述左腿受伤，护士检查伤口出血，有压痛，故选 C。

4. B　病人右臂关节痛，活动受限，有关节炎的可能，故选 B。

5. E　病人剧烈咳嗽、胸痛、发烧、呼吸困难，可能患了肺炎，故选 E。

Part Two

6. A　起初病人胃痛，后转移到右下腹，故本句正确。

7. B　根据对话，病人只是感到恶心，并不呕吐，故本句错。

8. A　护士量了病人的体温，发现他发低烧。本句正确。

9. B　护士让病人别紧张，说明病人开始时紧张，故本句错。

10. A　医生检查后，护士告诉病人患了阑尾炎，必须手术，还让病人签署手术知情同意书，病人同意合作，故本句正确。

Part Three

11. B　病人认为针灸非常了不起(really great)，故选 B。

12. A　中医理论中，疾病来自于人体内阴阳的不协调，故选 A。

13. C　按照中医理论，治疗疾病就是重新建立(reestablishment) 阴阳的平衡，故选 C。

14. B　阴阳之间的关系是对立的双方，故选 B。

15. C　与西医相比，中医在治疗神经系统疾病方面的优势是不会有副作用，故选 C。

Part Four

16. Tweedie　根据病人回答以及医生确认的拼写来确定。

17. tripped and fell　病人回答是绊倒造成的伤口。

18. wrapped a bandage　病人自述妻子给自己包扎止血。

19. a local anesthesia　病人会被施以局部麻醉止痛，以便于缝针。

20. anti-tetanus　病人需要重新注射抗破伤风药物。

Ⅱ Reading and Writing

Part One

21. C　可以利用 self-affirming 快速找到原文 C 段中的文字，即“This successful experience causes self-affirming thoughts, which boost our self-esteem, make us feel good, and lead us to believe we will do well in the future.”

22. D　基于 natural growth process 比较容易查到原文 D 段信息“This is, however, an equally powerful downward spiral that can interrupt the natural growth process.”从“however, downward, interrupt”可以推断本段说的是与前面相反的情况。

23. A 第3题题干是原文A段信息的变化表述:In a broader sense, people with an optimistic view of themselves outperform those who are doubtful or simply more "realistic"...

24. D 可以从 fail 一词大致定位,快速查到原文D段"When we fail, we say 'I told you so' to ourselves and make a mental note to avoid similar situations in the future."

25. E 根据本题题干中的 the authority figures 可以找到原文E段"The authority figures in our lives often shape our early thoughts and feelings."

26. F 本题句子较短,可凭借短期记忆整句寻找;或仅根据 play out(进行、开展,实施)查找。

27. B 从题干 learning to see yourself as a winner 可以找到本题位于原文B段:"Learning to see yourself as a winner and to feel like a winner happens primarily as a result of having successful experiences and thinking self-affirming thoughts."

28. E 本题题干的意思与原文E段第二句话的意思一致:"The authority figures in our lives often shape our early thoughts and feelings."

29. D 本题题干亦较短,整句寻找并不困难,其位于D段第三句:"We feel anxious about our performance and we avoid or remove ourselves from anxiety-producing situations."

30. B 本题题干说的是乐观积极的态度,而原文B段整段表达的都是乐观积极的态度,可初步得以定位;然后很容易便能查找到第三句"When we believe our efforts will be successful, we are more likely to undertake an activity or task."

Part Two

31. A 根据文章第二段,其研究的目的是"... to find out why otherwise healthy farmers ... appeared to be losing their ability to think and reason at a relatively early age ..."

32. B 本题题干为 one thousand old people,而原文第三段则是 a thousand people of different ages and various occupations,故本题错。

33. B 参照第五段原文"Contraction of front and side parts ... was observed in some subjects in their thirties."题干中的 shrink 与原文的 contraction 同义,所以两者表述相反,故本题错。

34. B 原文第五段第一句"... was observed in some subjects in their thirties"中为 some subjects,与题干 all the subjects 相悖;且原文 but 后的文字与题干意思亦相左。

35. B 第七段第二句"Those least at risk, says Matsuzawa, are lawyers ..."意为"脑萎缩出现在律师身上的机率最小"。

36. A 第四段结尾"The rear section of the brain ... does not contract with age ..."与题干意思一致。

37. A 参照第四段首句"... the front and side sections of the brain, which are related to intellect and emotion and determine the human character."这里关键是找准 which 从句的先行词。

38. B 第七段末句"White collar workers ... are ... as likely to have shrinking brains as

farm workers ... ”与题干意思相反。

39. B 参照第七段首句“... contraction of the brain begins sooner in people in the country than in the town. ”题干与原文表述刚好相反。

40. C 参照结尾段“... thinking can prevent the brain from shrinking. ”“The best way to maintain good blood circulation is through using the brain. ”该段指出，用脑是防止脑萎缩的最佳途径，但并未断言是唯一的方法。

Part Three

41. A 文章开头“People in the past did not question the difference between life and death. ”意为过去人们并未对生与死的区别提出过质疑，说明生与死的区别对他们而言很简单；又根据首段第5句“Today the difference between life and death is not as easy to see as in the past”，可以判断过去人们判断生与死很简单。

42. B 定位第一段第三句“... the body does not die immediately when the heart stops beating. ”此句与选项B之意正好相反。

43. A 定位第二段首句“This question has caused much debate among citizens in the United States. ”选项A中的“heated argument”对应此处的“much debate”。

44. C 答案C可定位于第三段开头两句：“The brain is made of thousands of millions of nerve cells. These cells send and receive millions of chemical and electrical messages every day. In this way the brain controls the other body activities. ”

45. C 末段尾句指出，“... the idea of brain wave activity as a test of death is slowly being accepted. ”与题干“Gradually more and more people begin to accept ... ”意思相近；而选项C中“the brain stops working”，意即大脑死亡，则对应原文中大脑停止活动即为死亡这一观点。

Part Four

46. F 根据原文第三句“Medical experts say ... . ”可知，处理伤口的第一步为用清水清理伤口，这与选项F“To clean the area around the wound, experts suggest using a clean cloth and soap. They say there is no need to use products like hydrogen peroxide or iodine. ”所表达的意思具有逻辑上的前后关系。

47. C 原文第五句是“It is important to remove all dirt and other material from the wound. ”而选项C正好是其承接语：“After the wound is cleaned ... ”

48. D 原文第7句“... these medicated products can ... ”谈的是这些产品的功效，而选项D“They also help to ... ”是唯一也谈产品功效的选项。

49. A 原文第9句提及bandage，而备选项中与bandage有关的选项只有A。

50. B 原文第11句谈signs of infection，而选项B“A high body temperature is also a sign of infection. ”与其内容吻合。

Part Five

51. E 此处为不定式，应该使用动词原形；再从句首的Hand washing及句末的the spread of disease可以判断空处应该为“预防”的意思。

52. D 从本空前的the most及空格后的名词ways来看，此空应推断为形容词。选项D effective为形容词，且其词义符合句意。

53. G　此空前是不定式 to reduce，其后为名词 diseases，故能较容易地推断出此空应填一形容词，唯有 G infectious 合乎要求。

54. C　get 对应上文的 touch，联系上句的 germs，此处应该仍然指细菌，只是换一个词表达而已。

55. L　or 一词表明空处所缺之词与其后的 coughed 相对应，L sneezed 从词义及动词形式均合乎要求。

56. I　"... food __ by ..."说明空处为动词的过去分词作后置定语，所以用 prepared。

57. H　本空所在句子说的是常识问题：接触钱后要洗手；且介词 after 后需用动名词，故 H touching 符合要求。

58. B　此空或是全文最容易的一空，因其要求填写的 defense 一词已出现在文章的标题中，只要读过标题，便很容易确定。

59. A　根据本句的句意应能推断出此空应为"传播"之意。

60. J　此句意思十分明确，空格处应填 wash 一类的词，故选 J rinse。

Part Six

61.

A Case Report

James Brown, a 26-month-old boy, was admitted to the hospital on July 5, 2014. His parents complained that he had been crying for two days.

Signs and symptoms of the boy include: a high temperature of 41.2℃, excessive mucus in nose and throat, rash on neck and shoulders, having difficulty in breathing, and vomit once every another hour. Diagnosis shows that the baby is under the condition of dehydration.

Major nursing instructions for him are as follows: a) The boy should have much drink. b) A lukewarm sponge bath is favored for the baby. c) During daytime the baby only needs to wear light bedclothes.

【审题】

这是一篇关于病例报告的写作。要求考生写不少于 100 词，内容应包括：病人姓名、年龄、入院时间、症状、诊断、医嘱等。表格中的信息要尽量表述完整，无遗漏；但也要注意不要超词太多。考生应注意使用常见的表达用语，如：be admitted to the hospital /be hospitalized; signs and symptoms of the patient include ...; as follows 等。

【范文评述】

本篇范文内容详实，涵盖了试题中提供的所有细节，包括病人的症状、诊断及医嘱等。语言通顺，无病句或其他语法错误。在时态的使用方面也十分妥帖，如第一段主要用过去时，因陈述过去的事实，如入院时间、主诉等；而第二、三两段则主要使用一般现在时，因其内容为病人症状及医嘱。在语言使用上也有可圈可点之处，如：第二段的 include 后的宾语均为名词性短语，而第三段的注意事项则均用完整的句子表达。

医护英语水平考试(二级)

模拟训练(二)

听力文本

This is METS-2 listening test. There are four parts in the test, Parts One, Two, Three, and Four. You will hear each part twice. Now, look at the instructions for Part One.
You will hear five patients describing their problems. Decide what problem each patient has. Write the appropriate letter A-H in each box. Mark the corresponding letter on your answer sheet. You will hear each conversation twice.
Here is an example:
Nurse (Woman): Good morning. What seems to be your problem?
Patient (Man): I have a pain in my stomach.
Nurse (Woman): Did you vomit?
Patient (Man): No, I didn't.
The answer is stomachache, so write letter F in the box. Now we are ready to start.

Conversation 1

Nurse (Woman): What's the matter with you, Peter?
Patient (Man): I have red spots all over my body.
Nurse (Woman): Do you have a fever?
Patient (Man): Yes, I do. This morning my temperature was 39 degrees.
Nurse (Woman): Well, according to the symptoms, you may have the measles.

Conversation 2

Nurse (Woman): What seems to be the problem, Mr. Jones?
Patient (Man): I'm suffering from insomnia.
Nurse (Woman): How long have you had this problem?
Patient (Man): Three months.
Nurse (Woman): Have you taken any medicine?
Patient (Man): I tried some sleeping pills, but they have done nothing for me.

Conversation 3

Nurse (Woman): You don't look well, Tim. What happened?
Patient (Man): Well, I fell off my bike and my left leg was wounded.
Nurse (Woman): Let me have a look. Oh, it's swollen and there is bruising. Does it hurt

when I press here?
Patient (Man): Yes, it hurts severely.
Nurse (Woman): OK. I'll get some iced water for you first.

Conversation 4

Nurse (Woman): Good morning. What's troubling you, William?
Patient (Man): Yesterday I had a running nose. Now my nose is stuffed up. I have a sore throat. And I'm afraid I've got a fever, too. I feel terrible.
Nurse (Woman): Don't worry, young man. Let me give you an examination. Open your mouth and say "ah".
Patient (Man): Ah.
Nurse (Woman): Your throat is inflamed. And your tongue is thickly coated. You have all the symptoms of influenza.

Conversation 5

Nurse (Woman): How are you? Mr. Hockings, what brings you to the clinic today?
Patient (Man): I am just feeling really tired lately.
Nurse (Woman): How long have you been feeling this way?
Patient (Man): About six weeks.
Nurse (Woman): Have you had any chest pain?
Patient (Man): Just very slightly.

This is the end of Part One. Now look at Part Two. You will hear a conversation between a patient and a nurse before an operation. For each of the following sentences, decide whether it is True (A) or False (B). Put a tick (√) in the relevant box. Mark the corresponding letter on your answer sheet. You will hear the conversation twice.

Nurse (Woman): Hello, I'm Wendy. I'm a theater nurse and I'm going to check you in today. How are you doing?
Patient (Man): All right.
Nurse (Woman): That's good. I'm just going to go through this checklist again. OK? Um, I know you've already answered many of these questions, but we like to do double-check everything, OK?
Patient (Man): Yes, that's fine.
Nurse (Woman): Right, can you tell me your full name, please?
Patient (Man): Yes, John Smith.
Nurse (Woman): Thank you. I'll have a quick look at your identification bracelets if I may?
Patient (Man): Sure, here they are.

Nurse (Woman): John Smith, bed number six seven four nine. Can you tell me what operation you're having today?
Patient (Man): Yes, I'm having the tendon in my right shoulder repaired.
Nurse (Woman): Mm, did you sign a consent form for the operation?
Patient (Man): Yes, I did.
Nurse (Woman): All right, nearly finished. Have you had any pre-operative medicine?
Patient (Man): Yes, I had an injection just before I came here.
Nurse (Woman): Mm, pre-med given and signed for. Great. All right, I'll sign the checklist and you've already got a theater cap to cover your hair. You'll be waiting here for a few more minutes and then we'll take you through. Are you all right?
Patient (Man): Yes, thanks.

This is the end of Part Two. Now look at Part Three. You will hear a conversation between Patrica, a doctor, and Paul, a patient, about his discomforts. For each of the following questions or unfinished sentences, choose the correct answer A, B or C. Put a tick (√) in the relevant box. Mark the corresponding letter on your answer sheet. You will hear the conversation twice.
Doctor (Woman): Hello, Paul. How are you feeling now?
Patient (Man): Oh, not too good. Everything hurts.
Doctor (Woman): Mm, I can imagine. You've got a lot of cuts and bruises. Can you tell me where the pain is?
Patient (Man): Yeah. My head, my cheek ... um, the broken cheek, I mean. My arms hurt where the cuts are and my chest hurts, too.
Doctor (Woman): OK. Can you tell me if the pain is the same all over or different?
Patient (Man): I've got a throbbing headache, and my right cheek hurts when I touch it.
Doctor (Woman): What about the pain in your arms and chest?
Patient (Man): It's a stinging pain in the shallow cuts, but this cut in my chest is quite deep, and the pain's sharp like a knife.
Doctor (Woman): When does the pain get worse?
Patient (Man): It's worse when I turn over or move.
Doctor (Woman): OK, can you rate the pain for me? On a scale of zero to ten, zero is when you feel no pain and ten is when you feel the worst pain that you can imagine. What's the pain like now when you are at rest?
Patient (Man): It's around six.
Doctor (Woman): And when you move a bit?
Patient (Man): It gets worse. Seven, at least.
Doctor (Woman): All right, I'll get you some painkillers. Is there anything else which relieves the pain?
Patient (Man): One nurse gave me a heat pack for my chest, and that helped.

Doctor (Woman): All right. I'll put you in a comfortable position with some more pillows and get you a heat pack, too.
Patient (Man): Thanks. It's hard for me to sleep when I'm in pain.
Doctor (Woman): I'll pull the curtains around and dim the lights a bit for you.

This is the end of Part Three. Now look at Part Four. You will hear a conversation between a doctor and a patient in the outpatient department. Fill in the blanks. Write the answers on your answer sheet. You will hear the conversation twice.
Nurse (Woman): Sir, have you registered yet?
Patient (Man): No, I haven't.
Nurse (Woman): Do you have your history sheet?
Patient (Man): Yes, here you are.
Nurse (Woman): Now let's fill this admission card. What's your name?
Patient (Man): Wentworth Connolly. C-O-N-N-O-L-L-Y.
Nurse (Woman): Your marriage, age and profession?
Patient (Man): I am married, 28 years old and I'm an engineer.
Nurse (Woman): Oh, let me see. Now your hospital number is 453789.
Patient (Man): Thanks.
Nurse (Woman): How long do you expect to stay in the hospital?
Patient (Man): The doctor told me to stay for about one month. I have nephritis. This is my second time to enter the hospital. I found blood in my urine and my blood pressure is 140/90.
Nurse (Woman): Would you come to the hospital today?
Patient (Man): Yes, I hope to enter the hospital this morning.
Nurse (Woman): But there is no bed available now. This afternoon, two patients will be discharged. So you may be admitted then.
Patient (Man): Well, when they leave the hospital, I shall be admitted. By the way, when are the visiting hours?
Nurse (Woman): The visiting hours are from 9 to 11 o'clock in the morning and 3 to 5 in the afternoon.
Patient (Man): Thank you for introducing the information. Good bye.
Nurse (Woman): Good bye. See you in the afternoon.
This is the end of Part Four. You now have five minutes to write your answers on the answer sheet. You have one more minute. This is the end of the listening test.

参考答案及解析

Ⅰ Listening

Part One

1. D 本题中护士根据症状判断诊断可能为荨麻疹(measles),故选 D。

2. G 本题中病人自述失眠(insomnia),故选 G。

3. C 本题中护士通过检查发现患者腿部淤青(bruising),故选 C。

4. E 本题中护士根据患者一系列症状判断其患有流感(influenza),故选 E。

5. B 本题中病人自述乏力(tired),故选 B。

Part Two

6. B 护士提及"I'm just going to go through this checklist again."关键词 again 提示这不是第一次核对检查表,故本句错。

7. B 病人自述"I'm having the tendon in my right shoulder repaired."而不是左肩,故本句错。

8. B 当护士询问患者是否已经签手术同意书时,患者明确肯定回答。故本句错。

9. A 患者自述"I had an injection just before I came here",故本句正确。

10. A 护士快速检查了患者的 identification bracelets(身份识别腕带)并核对床号"bed number six seven four nine",故本句正确。

Part Three

11. C 患者讲述到疼痛的部位有头部(head)、面颊(cheek)、臂膀(arm)和胸部(chest),故选 C。

12. B 患者自述浅切口的疼痛"It's a stinging pain in the shallow cuts",故选 B。

13. A 医生让患者衡量疼痛等级,患者回答"around six",故选 A。

14. A 医生问患者疼痛何时变得更严重,患者回答"when I move",故选 A。

15. C 医生为了减缓患者疼痛,给以止痛药 painkillers 及热敷袋 a heat pack,故选 C。

Part Four

16. 28/twenty-eight 患者回答年龄 28 岁。

17. One month 患者谈话中提及需住院大约一个月时间。

18. engineer 患者回答职业工程师。

19. Blood 患者自述病情时提及"I found blood in my urine ..."。

20. 140/90 患者自述病情时提及"... and my blood pressure is 140/90."

Ⅱ Reading and Writing

Part One

21. B 可以利用 rash, itching, asthma 快速找到原文 B 段中的文字,即"Responses may include itching, redness or tearing of the eyes, skin rash, asthma, sneezing, and urticaria."

22. C　可以利用关键词 surgical operation，快速查找原文 C 段中的文字，即“An inflamed appendix is usually surgically removed ...”

23. D　可以利用关键词 damage to muscle and connective tissues 快速查找原文 D 段中的文字，即“... but it probably involves damage to muscle and connective tissues.”

24. B　可以利用关键词 an overreaction of the immune system，快速查找原文 B 段中的文字，即“It is a harmful overreaction by the immune system ...”

25. A　通过 iron-deficiency anemia 快速查找原文 A 段中的文字，即“The most common type of anemia is iron-deficiency anemia caused by ...”

26. C　利用关键词 pain 排除几个疾病，然后进一步利用 pain shift，确定答案为 C。

27. A　利用 fatigue，palpitation，shortness of breath 这三个关键词，快速查找原文 A 段中的文字，即“The general symptoms include fatigue，shortness of breath，heart palpitation and irritability.”

28. E　通过关键词 proper rest and nutrition 快速查找原文 E 段中的文字，即“With proper rest and nutrition，the body can correct the problem，and cramping stops.”

29. C　利用关键词 fever，nausea，vomiting and appetite loss 这四个症状，快速查找原文 C 段中的文字，即“A lower-grade fever may be present along with nauseated vomiting and loss of appetite.”

30. F　通过关键词 blood glucose 快速查找原文 F 段中的文字，即“It's characterized by constant high levels of blood glucose (sugar).”

Part Two

31. A　根据文章第一段“The most common symptoms are diarrhea，vomiting and stomach pain，because whatever causes the condition inflames the gastrointestinal tract.”故本题对。

32. A　根据文章第一段“... because whatever causes the condition inflames the gastrointestinal tract.”故本题对。

33. A　根据文章第二段“Bacterial infection is frequently a factor，and infection by parasites can cause acute gastroenteritis to last for several weeks. Viruses can also cause lengthy stomach flu.”故本题对。

34. B　定位第二段 Bacteria，parasites，virus can cause gastroenteritis. 再根据医学常识和上下文判断应该 parasite 是“寄生虫”，不属于细菌，故本题错。

35. B　根据文章第三段“Some types of acute gastroenteritis will not resolve without antibiotic treatment，especially when bacteria or exposure to parasites are the cause.”故本题错。

36. C　文中没有提到。

37. A　参照文章第四段最后一句：“Dehydration can actually cause greater nausea，and even organ shutdown if not properly addressed.”故本题对。

38. B　参照文章第五段第二句：“Generally，contact with the fecal matter of a person with the condition and then improperly washing or not washing the hands causes acute gastroenteritis to be quite contagious.”故本题错。

39. A 参照文章第五段第二句："... then improperly washing or not washing the hands causes acute gastroenteritis to be quite contagious."故本题对。

40. B 参照文章第六段第一句："Other methods of transmission of acute gastroenteritis can include eating food or drinking liquids contaminated with bacteria or parasites."故本题错。

Part Three

41. C 根据"After cutting through the skin"定位在文章第二段，介绍手术过程，然后通过 the bladder and uterus exposed，迅速找到原文"After cutting through the skin, fat, and muscle of the abdomen, the membrane that covers the internal organs is opened, exposing the bladder and uterus."

42. C 根据"after the procedure"定位在文章第三段，迅速找到原文"The mother is allowed to recover for approximately three to five days in the hospital."

43. B 本题是关于"在何种情况下需要剖腹产"，所以定位在文章的第一段第二句"Under conditions of fetal distress, or in the case of breech presentation (when a baby is turned feet at the time of delivery), or if the woman's first baby was born by Cesarean delivery, a procedure called a Cesarean section may be required."以及最后一句"Many are also performed upon request."

44. A 通过关键词 lateral incision 迅速定位在第二段，然后找到原句"... a doctor will make either a lateral incision in the skin just above the pubic hair line, or a vertical incision below the naval."

45. A 本题是关于剖腹产手术步骤的，涉及文章第二、三段。通过 at the beginning; when the bladder and uterus are exposed; at the end of a Cesarean 这三个短语，对应相应的手术步骤，然后再根据原文中 Many are also performed upon request 判断 A 选项是正确的。

Part Four

46. B 讲述静脉输液流程步骤，前面已准备输液袋并洗手，此处应核查药品、医嘱和输液单的一致。

47. C 讲述静脉输液流程步骤，准备输液管与输液器。

48. A 讲述静脉输液流程的步骤，调节滴速。

49. E 讲述静脉输液流程的步骤，给病人扎针。

50. D 讲述静脉输液流程的步骤，填写输液单和体液平衡表。

Part Five

51. B help 后接动词原形，而且根据句意"帮助鉴别疼痛的原因"，故选 B。

52. L 不定式后接动词原形，而且根据句意"分娩教育是处理问题的一个好的方法。"故选 L。

53. K will 后接动词原形，根据句意"分娩教育是处理问题的一个好的方法，但却无法彻底解决这一问题"，故选 K。

54. I 根据语法，这里需要动词的第三人称单数，因为主语是 this。再根据冒号后列举的四项 reading, touring birth facility, discussion with care providers and numerous other

sources of information,最终确定选 I。

55. A 根据语法,这里缺的是动词的现在分词形式,再根据句意,故选 A。

56. D 根据语法,介词后面接动词的现在分词形式,再根据句意,故选 D。

57. J 根据句意,Certain positions 后一定是介绍某种手术体位的,再根据 on your back,所以确定是平躺姿势,故选 J。

58. C 根据语法,这里需要一个形容词,再根据句意,故选 C。

59. H 根据本句话的含义,"这不会发生在每个人身上",故选 H。

60. F 根据语法,这里需要一个动词原形。而且根据动词后面的 the baby to turn 判断出这个动词后可以接 to do sth.,故选 F。

Part Six

61.

Discharge Summary

John Davis was hospitalized with a complaint of nausea and vomiting for nearly one month. Examination of the abdomen showed that there were some bowel sounds. He was diagnosed with acute gastroenteritis and chronic non-atrophic gastritis.

The patient was admitted on October 7, 2008 and had mineral supplement. The patient's condition got improved, showing gradual resolution of nausea and vomiting. The patient was discharged on October 12, 2008 in stable condition.

The result of the treatment is very good and the patient turned for the better quickly. No medications are needed after discharge. But if this patient cannot get used to Chinese food, he had better return to the UK as soon as possible to prevent the relapse of acute gastroenteritis. Since he doesn't have immediate family members in China and he lives a quite independent life, it is suggested that he be visited by nurses twice a month.

【审题】

这是一篇关于出院小结的写作。要求考生写 100 字左右的简要的出院记录,内容应包括:病人姓名、年龄、入院时间、症状、诊断、医嘱等。考生须注意格式与表达;表格中的信息要尽量表述完整,无遗漏;语言表达尽量简明扼要,不能超词,并适当运用一些专业的术语和表达方式。

【范文评述】

本篇范文内容详实,涵盖了试题中提供的绝大部分细节,包括病人的症状、诊断治疗及出院医嘱等。语言通顺,无病句或其他语法错误。在内容安排方面,第一段主要陈述患者入院前情况,包括入院时间、原因等;而第二段主要陈述住院期间治疗情况;第三段讲述出院后患者医嘱与注意事项。在语言使用上用语准确地道,句型符合规范,是一篇不错的范文。

医护英语水平考试(二级)

模拟训练(三)

听力文本

This is METS-2 listening test. There are four parts in the test, Parts One, Two, Three, and Four. You will hear each part twice. Now, look at the instructions for Part One.
You will hear five conversations about effects of some medications. Write the appropriate letter A-G in each box. Mark the corresponding letter on your answer sheet. You will hear each conversation twice.
Here is an example:
Patient (Man): Doctor, I'm always worried about bone loss. What should I do?
Doctor (Woman): Why not take this kind of medication? It can prevent skeletal diseases that weaken bones.
The answer is to prevent skeletal diseases, so write letter F in the box. Now we are ready to start.

Conversation 1

Patient (Man): Doctor, can you tell me how I take this kind of medicine?
Doctor (Woman): You should take two capsules after meals, three times a day.
Patient (Man): Why did you prescribe it for me?
Doctor (Woman): Well, this medicine has wide anti-bacteria property which can alleviate the signs of your inflammation.

Conversation 2

Patient (Man): Doctor, what's the name of the medication in my prescription?
Doctor (Woman): Let me have a look. Oh, it is called Vitamin E.
Patient (Man): What's its function? Are there any side effects?
Doctor (Woman): It contains many antioxidants and may slower the process of skin wrinkling. We haven't found any side effects at present. Don't worry about that!

Conversation 3

Patient (Man): Excuse me, Nurse. Would you please tell me something about this medicine?
Nurse (Woman): My pleasure. This medicine is for patients with asthma.
Patient (Man): What about its function?.

Nurse (Woman) According to the instruction on the bottle, it can reduce sputum production.

Conversation 4

Patient (Man): Nurse, how should I take these white tablets?
Nurse (Woman): You'd better take them on empty stomach.
Patient (Man): Why should I take them?
Nurse (Woman): Well, they are very effective to relieve your pain.

Conversation 5

Patient (Man): Doctor, I need your help.
Doctor (Woman): My pleasure. What's the trouble?
Patient (Man): I can't tell from these bottles.
Doctor (Woman): Don't worry. Oh, these are for IV drip. They can help to balance your body fluid.

This is the end of Part One. Now look at Part Two. You will hear a conversation between a patient and a nurse about his appendicitis. For each of the following sentences, decide whether it is True (A) or False (B). Put a tick (√) in the relevant box. Mark the corresponding letter on your answer sheet. You will hear the conversation twice.

Patient (Man): Nurse, I'm not feeling well today.
Nurse (Woman): Where don't you feel well?
Patient (Man): I have a pain in my abdomen.
Nurse (Woman): How long have you had it?
Patient (Man): It started in the morning. At the beginning I had a stomachache.
Nurse (Woman): How long did it last?
Patient (Man): About 3 hours, but this afternoon it moved to the right lower part of the abdomen for 5 hours.
Nurse (Woman): Have you had any vomiting?
Patient (Man): I have only nausea.
Nurse (Woman): Have you any diarrhea?
Patient (Man): No.
Nurse (Woman): Any fever?
Patient (Man): I don't know.
Nurse (Woman): Let me take your temperature. All right, you have a slight fever.
Nurse (Woman): Please lie down on the bed; loosen your belt, please. Let the doctor examine your abdomen.
Patient (Man): Thank you.

Nurse (Woman): Don't be nervous and try to relax.

Patient (Man): All right.

Nurse (Woman): The result of your blood test tells us that your white blood cell count is 18,000. The doctor said that you had acute appendicitis.

Patient (Man): Oh, I am scared.

Nurse (Woman): Don't be afraid, you will recover. The doctor said that you have to have an operation. So, please sign your name on the consent form to say that you agree to the doctor operation on you.

Patient (Man): I'll cooperate.

Nurse (Woman): Thanks for your cooperation.

This is the end of Part Two. Now look at Part Three. You will hear a conversation between a patient and a doctor about treatment of eyes. For questions 11 - 15, choose the correct answer A, B or C. Put a tick (√) in the box. You will hear the conversation twice.

Patient (Man): Doctor, I have sore eyes for three days. Could you give me an examination?

Doctor (Woman): All right. Your eyes have been red. Have you had any problems with your eyes before?

Patient (Man): No, I haven't.

Doctor (Woman): I'll examine your eyes first. The sight is normal. Any other troubles except the red and sore eyes?

Patient (Man): I feel an itch in my eyes as if there was something in them. There is much secretion from the eyes, and they also fear light a little.

Doctor (Woman): Let me have a look. You have acute injective conjunctivitis. You require some treatment.

Patient (Man): What can you give me for it?

Doctor (Woman): First, you'll have your eyes irrigated. You will feel a little pain when I irrigate the eyes. Don't be afraid. I think you can stand it. It will help cure your problems.

Patient (Man): What should I pay attention to?

Doctor (Woman): You must put the eyedrops and ointment into your eyes on time, once half an hour. This kind of disease is infectious and it is necessary to pay attention to isolation. Your basin and towel should be separated from those of others and they also should be sterilized regularly. Wash your hands before and after instilling the drops in your eyes. Wipe your eyes with a clean handkerchief. Don't go to the public places. Don't touch others' things. It will protect both you and others. Don't cover the eyes or use hot compress, otherwise it will be helpful for the germs to develop and breed. Come here everyday to have your eyes irrigated. If you do what I tell you, you will soon be well again.

Patient (Man): Thank you, doctor.

Doctor (Woman): You're welcome.

This is the end of Part Three. Now look at Part Four. You will hear a doctor persuading a patient. Listen and complete questions 16 - 20 on your answer sheet. You will hear the conversation twice.

Doctor (Man): Well, Mrs. Wilkins, what you've got in your breast is a lump of fibrosis tissue. No real cause for worrying, but I think we should deal with it.

Patient (Woman): Oh, is it serious?

Doctor (Man): No, it's not, but it won't get better of its own accord. I'd recommend you to come in and will deal with the situation by operation.

Patient (Woman): Couldn't the lump be melted away by medicine?

Doctor (Man): Sorry, I don't think so. An operation is the only way to stop the problem.

Patient (Woman): Oh, dear. It's not cancer, is it?

Doctor (Man): No, it's not cancer, but I think you will be a lot more comfortable without the tumor there.

Patient (Woman): I suppose you know best, but I'm frightened of hospitals.

Doctor (Man): I know, but hospitals are useful places to turn to when you need them. You'll only be in for ten days or so, and once the operation is over, you'll feel so much better. Shall I put you on the waiting list?

Patient (Woman): I suppose so. How long will it be?

Doctor (Man): Hard to tell it exactly, but about 6 weeks. Is that all right for your holidays?

Patient (Woman): Yes, let's get it over with before then.

Doctor (Man): Very well, Mrs. Wilkins. We'll wait for you to get this fixed up. Goodbye, and don't worry about hospitals.

Patient (Woman): Goodbye, doctor, and thanks very much.

This is the end of Part Four. You now have five minutes to write your answers on the answer sheet. You have one more minute. This is the end of the listening test.

参考答案及解析

Ⅰ Listening

Part One

1. C　医生描述该药物可以减轻炎症症状(... which can alleviate the signs of your inflammation),故选 C。

2. E　医生介绍药物为维生素 E,可减缓皮肤起皱,故选 E。

3. D　护士介绍该药物能减少痰液,对哮喘病人有效,故选 D。

4. A　护士让病人空腹服用该药物,说这些药片能减轻疼痛,故选 A。

5. G　医生介绍该药用于静脉滴注,能平衡病人的体液,故选 G。

Part Two

6. A　此句意思是:病人腹痛。根据对话,起初病人胃痛,后转移到右下腹,故本句正确。

7. B　此句意思是:病人呕吐了几个小时。根据对话,病人只是感到恶心,并没呕吐,故本句错。

8. A　此句意思是:护士给病人量了体温,发现他有低热。对话中护士说要量一下体温,结果发现他发低烧。故本句正确。

9. B　此句意思是:病人在腹部检查时很放松。对话中,护士让病人别紧张,说明病人开始时是紧张的,故本句错误。

10. A　此句意思是:病人得了阑尾炎,将接受手术治疗。对话中,护士告诉病人医生的检查结果是阑尾炎,必须手术,还让病人签署手术知情同意书,病人同意合作,故本句正确。

Part Three

11. C　题干的意思是:病人眼疾的症状不包括哪一项。根据病人自述 I have sore eyes for three days,医生观察后说 Your eyes have been red,检查后称 The sight is normal,故选 C。

12. A　题干的意思是:病人的感觉是什么。根据对话,病人感觉到眼部发痒(an itch in my eyes),眼中有大量的分泌物(much secretion from the eyes),轻微畏光(fear light a little),故选 A。

13. A　题干的意思是:按照医生的建议,病人应该做什么。对话中医生要求病人使用滴眼液和眼药膏每半小时一次(once half an hour,即每小时两次),由于该眼疾有传染性需要注意隔离,故选 A。

14. B　题干的意思是:按照医生的建议,病人不应该做什么。对话中医生告诉病人不能遮盖眼部或使用热敷,故选 B。

15. C　题干的意思是:什么对细菌的繁殖有利。对话中医生告诉病人不能遮盖眼部或使用热敷,否则将有利于细菌繁殖(otherwise it will be helpful for the germs to develop and breed)。由此判断遮盖眼睛或热敷有助于细菌繁殖,故选 C。

Part Four

16. Mrs. Wilkins　根据对话中两次提到的病人名字填写。

17. breast 根据医生的陈述 What you've got in your breast 来填写。

18. tissue 根据医生的陈述 a lump of fibrosis tissue 来填写。

19. medicine 根据病人问话 Couldn't the lump be melted away by medicine? 来确定。

20. operation 对话中医生两次说到用手术来解决问题。

Ⅱ Reading and Writing

Part One

21. D 利用关键词 extreme stress 推测是儿童虐待的身心影响,找到应属部分 D 段开头的 causes,然后查到原文"Extreme stress can impair the development of the nervous and immune systems."进行比对。

22. F 利用关键词 several risk factors 查找到 F 段原文:A number of risk factors for child maltreatment have been identified.

23. A 利用关键词 global estimates for the prevalence of child maltreatment 可以快速定位到 A 段,从而找到原句:There are no reliable global estimates for the prevalence of child maltreatment.

24. E 利用关键词 economic impact 可以判断出其所属段落讲的是儿童虐待的影响,从而快速定位到 E 段:Beyond the health consequences of child maltreatment, there is an economic impact, including ...

25. C 从 significant proportion of deaths 入手,可迅速找到 C 段原文:This number underestimates the true extent of the problem, as a significant proportion of deaths due to child maltreatment are ...

26. D 从 causes 判断应该在 D 段,进一步查找原文:Maltreatment causes stress that is associated with disruption in early brain development.

27. B 利用百分比数字 25%—50%可快速定位至 B 段,找到原文:... while 25%—50% of all children report being physically abused.

28. C 利用关键词 31,000 homicide deaths 可定位至 C 段,找到原文:Every year, there are estimated 31,000 homicide deaths in children under 15.

29. D 根据题干意思判断该句陈述的是儿童虐待对其身心的危害,所以定位 D 段,查找原文:maltreatment can contribute to heart disease, cancer, suicide and sexually transmitted infections.

30. B 利用关键词 emotional abuse 判断应该是讲儿童虐待的类型,一般在文章比较靠前的部分有介绍,但不会在开头提出问题的段落,进而找到 B 段中的原文:Additionally, many children are subject to emotional abuse.

Part Two

31. A 文章第一段最后一句提到北欧人知道适量日光对人体健康有好处。(they also know that a certain amount of sunshine is good for their bodies and general health.)

32. B 文章第二段第一句就指出,古希腊人知道利用日光可以治病(In ancient Greece people knew about the healing powers of the sun.),与题干意思正好相反。

33. A 根据文章第二段内容了解到，古希腊人知道日光可以治病，但后来这一知识失传了，直到19世纪末期才又有人开始研究日光对某些疾病的作用。由此可见，历史上很长一段时间内人们没有用日光来治病。故此句正确。

34. B 原文用 not only ... but also ... 表示并列，该题使用的是 not ... but ...（不是……而是……），故本题错。

35. A 文章的最后一段提到：如果得了肺结核，不恰当的日光浴可能十分有害(If, for example, tuberculosis is attacking the lungs, unwise sunbathing may do great harm.)，故此句正确。

36. B 利用 rays 一词找到第三段原文：the rays of the sun with the greatest healing power are the infra-red and ultra-violet rays。而题干的意思是只有红外线具有最强的治疗作用，故本题错。

37. A 通过关键词 ultra-violet rays 找到第三段中的原句：but ultra-violet rays are too easily lost in fog and the polluted air near industrial towns。

38. C 文章的主题是日光的治疗作用。虽然文章第三段提到"Dr. Roller found that sunlight, fresh air and good food cure a great many diseases."但整篇文章中并未提到令人愉快的环境(amiable environment)能治病，所以无法确定此句的对错。

39. A 根据关键词 Dr. Roller 可定为至第三段，并找到原句：He decided to start a school where sick children could be cured and at the same time continue to learn.

40. B 利用 Roller's pupils 查找到第三段原文：Although they wore hardly any clothes, Roller's pupils were seldom cold。注意句中 hardly 一词含否定意义，故学生们很少感冒的原因并不是他们衣服穿得多。

Part Three

41. C 参照第一段第三句：The weight may come from muscle, bone, fat and/ or body water.

42. B 参照第二段第三句：Factors that might tip the balance include your genetic makeup, overeating, eating high-fat foods and not being physically active. "tip the balance"意为"打破平衡"。

43. C 通过比较第三和第四段的数据可以得出结论：20—74岁的成年人中肥胖人数增长最多，故正确答案为C。

44. C 文章讲述的主要是肥胖带来的健康问题，且在文章的第五段明确提到：Being overweight or obese increases the risk of many diseases and health conditions, including ... 故可以推断出C是正确答案。

45. A 注意最后一段的陈述是针对肥胖患者而言：If you are obese, losing even 5 to 10 percent of your weight can delay or prevent some of these diseases.

Part Four

46. C 从第Ⅰ步"a suitable donor heart"以及第Ⅱ步"also called a beating heart cadaver"判断此处应该说的是 donor heart 的来源，故选C。

47. A 从第Ⅲ步的病人入院接受评估和术前用药可推断出下一句应为捐献的心脏被取出并检查是否合适，同时参考第Ⅴ步"Learning that a potential organ is unsuitable can

induce distress ... ”判断前一步讲的应该是心脏是否合适(suitable)的问题。故选 A。

48. F 从第Ⅶ步给病人用免疫抑制剂抗排斥来倒推出前一步应该也是对病人进行手术前的各项检测,故选 F。

49. B 根据前一句中的 the patient is taken to the ICU to recover 来判断,下面一句应该是讲述病人从麻醉中清醒后的情况,故选 B。

50. D 根据第Ⅹ步病人住院时间的长短取决于病人的身体状况来判断,下一句应该仍然是有关住院治疗的时间问题,故选 D。

Part Five

51. K 根据空格前的 The 和其后的 or allergic reaction 可知此处应填入与过敏反应有关的一个名词。紧接着下面就列举了各种过敏症状。所以应选 K(symptom)。

52. I 根据句子结构,that 引导的是定语从句,修饰先行词 food or drugs,that 在定语从句中作主语,而空格后是介词 with,因此判断空格处应填入动词。而能与 with 搭配的动词便是 interfere,故选 I。interfere with 表示“干扰,影响”。

53. G 根据前面的短语 injections of penicillin or other ... 判断此处的单词应为名词,且与 penicillin 有关。而 penicillin(青霉素)是一种药物,所以应选 G(drugs)。

54. H 首先根据空格前的 a person's 和空格后的 system 可判断出此处应填入形容词。又根据句意及医学常识可知,此处应该是免疫系统,故选 H(immune)。

55. A 首先根据空格前的 an 可判断出此处为一个以元音因素开头的名词。然后根据医学常识,导致过敏反应的物质被称为过敏原,因此选 A(allergen)。

56. F 首先根据空格前的 an 判断此处应该是以元音因素开头的一个单词,再根据空格后面的 response 判定此单词为形容词,从而确定选择 F(inflammatory)。inflammatory response 意为“炎症反应”。

57. D 首先根据空格前的 exist to 判断此处用动词原形,再根据句子的意思作出选择。句意为“有各种测试可以诊断过敏状况”,故选 D(diagnose)。

58. B 首先根据空格前的 many 和空格后的 test results 判断此处应填入一个形容词,再根据句意确定答案。positive test results 意为“阳性测试结果”,与句意相符,故选 B。

59. E 根据空格后面的 such as swelling 可以判断此处为一种症状或反应。因 symptom 已用过,故选择 E(reaction)。

60. C 根据此空格前的 for 可判断此处应填入名词,再根据文章的主题来判断,此处为过敏的治疗方法,故选 C(allergy)。

Part Six

61.

A Patient Report

John, a 26-year-old male patient, was admitted on 3rd April 2014 because of severe acute right upper abdominal pain, accompanied by the rigidity of abdominal muscle.

The patient complained of hunger-like pain occurring at night or after meals and food was of no use to reduce the pain. On examination, the patient had a positive occult blood test and decreased complete blood count. The examination indicates duodenal ulcer with perforation. On this diagnosis, he received an operation, and so far he is in a good condition.

The patient needs enough rest and sleep and he should return for a check-up in 20 days.

【作文审题】

这是一篇关于病人情况报告的作文。根据题中所给的病人情况记录表，病人的姓名、年龄、入院时间、入院时病人的症状与主诉、医生的检查、诊断和治疗措施、病人目前的状态以及医嘱等信息一目了然。因此，在撰写报告时应将上述表单中的信息准确无误地表述清楚，避免遗漏重要信息。同时还需注意单词的拼写、句子的结构和语法问题，字数按要求尽量控制在90—110字。

【范文评析】

范文将病人情况记录表中所提供的重要信息(如病人的姓名、年龄、入院时间、入院时病人的症状与病情主诉、医生的检查、诊断和治疗措施、病人目前的状态以及医嘱等)按时间顺序准确无误地进行了描述，语句通顺，用词得当，语言简练，前后连贯，条理清楚，符合医学英语写作习惯。此外，作文中无单词拼写错误，语法正确，句子结构完整，句式丰富多样(如较好地运用了同位语、被动语态、分词结构、介词短语等形式)。因此，范文完全符合病人情况报告的写作要求。

医护英语水平考试(二级)

模拟训练(四)

听力文本

This is METS-2 Listening Test. There are four parts in the test, Parts One, Two, Three, and Four. You will hear each part twice. Now, look at the instructions for Part One.

You will hear five patients describing their problems. Decide what problem each patient has. Write the appropriate letter A-H in each box. Mark the corresponding letter on your answer sheet. You will hear each conversation twice.

Here is an example:

Nurse (Woman): Good morning. What's wrong with you?

Patient (Man): I have a severe pain in my joints for more than one week.

Nurse (Woman): Does it become shaper in rainy days?

Patient (Man): Yes, that's right.

The answer is arthritis, so write letter D in the box.

Now we are ready to start.

Conversation 1

Nurse (Woman): How can I help you, Sir?
Patient (Man): I have a terrible headache.
Nurse (Woman): When did it begin?
Patient (Man): About a week ago.

Conversation 2

Nurse(Woman): What brought you to the emergency room?
Patient (Man): I've got awful pains in my belly, and I feel like throwing up all the time. I feel awful.
Nurse (Woman): How long have you had this pain?
Patient (Man): It started last night, up here, but this morning it's here, and it really hurts.
Nurse (Woman): Has it moved again?
Patient (Man): No, it's been steady for 2 hours.

Conversation 3

Nurse (Woman): How do you feel this morning?
Patient (Man): Awful. My left lung hurts quite a bit.
Nurse (Woman): Don't worry, the infection in your lungs will be fine after the treatment.
Patient (Man): Thanks, it's really painful. Can I have a cold drink, please?
Nurse (Woman): OK, but what you need now is a good rest.

Conversation 4

Nurse (Woman): Good morning, Mr. Morgan. How are you today?
Patient (Man): A little better than yesterday.
Nurse (Woman): Since you started insulin injection yesterday, you should know how to use the insulin pen. It's easy for you to learn.
Patient (Man): Right, well, I'll follow the instructions.

Conversation 5

Nurse (Woman): You look pale, Mrs. Wilson. What's your problem?
Patient (Man): I often feel dizzy these days and tired of doing everything.
Nurse (Woman): Where is your blood test report? What did it say? Let me see.
Patient (Man): Here you are.
Nurse (Woman): Oh my God! The result of your blood test tells us that your hemoglobin is 5g/dl! It's much lower than the normal level which is 11g/dl.

This is the end of Part One. Now look at Part Two.

You will hear a conversation between a patient and a nurse about the acute appendicitis. For each of the following sentences, decide whether it is True (A) or False (B). Put a tick (√) in the relevant box. Mark the corresponding letter on your answer sheet. You will hear the conversation twice.

Patient (Woman): Nurse, I'm not feeling well today.

Nurse (Man): Where don't you feel well?

Patient (Woman): I have a pain in my abdomen.

Nurse (Man): How long have you had it?

Patient (Woman): It started in the morning. At the beginning I have a stomachache.

Nurse (Man): How long did it last?

Patient (Woman): About 3 hours, but this afternoon it moved to the lower right part of the abdomen for 5 hours.

Nurse (Man): Have you had any vomiting?

Patient (Woman): I have only nausea.

Nurse (Man): Constipation?

Patient (Woman): Yes.

Nurse (Man): Have you any diarrhea?

Patient (Woman): No.

Nurse (Man): Any fever?

Patient (Woman): I don't know.

Nurse (Man): Let me take your temperature. All right, you have a slight fever.

Nurse (Man): Please lie down on the bed. Loosen your belt, please. Let the doctor examine your abdomen.

Patient (Woman): Thank you.

Nurse (Man): Don't be nervous and try to relax.

Patient (Woman): All right.

Nurse (Man): The doctor said you need to collect a specimen of blood and urine for examination.

Patient (Woman): Yes.

Nurse (Man): The result of your blood test tells us that your white blood cell count is $18 * 10^9/L$.

Patient (Woman): I see. Thank you.

Nurse (Man): The doctor said that you had acute appendicitis.

Patient (Woman): Oh, gosh.

Nurse (Man): Don't be afraid. You will recover. The doctor said that you have to have an operation. So, please sign your name on the consent form to say that you agree to the operation on you.

Patient (Woman): I'll cooperate.

Nurse (Man): Thank you for your cooperation.

This is the end of Part Two. Now look at Part Three.

You will hear a conversation between a patient and a nurse about post-operative care. For each of the following questions or unfinished sentences, choose the correct answer A, B or C. Put a tick (√) in the relevant box. Mark the corresponding letter on your answer sheet. You will hear the conversation twice.

Nurse(Woman): Mr. Jones, how are you feeling today?

Patient (Man): Terrible. Why did you get me out of bed today? I just had surgery yesterday.

Nurse(Woman): It can prevent complications.

Patient (Man): I've never heard of that. When my dad had surgery, he was in bed for a week.

Nurse(Woman): They used to do that. Now we know that getting up early is better.

Patient (Man): But it hurts. And I feel dizzy.

Nurse(Woman): You were given a pain shot an hour before you got up. You should get up slowly. Look ahead and don't look down; you will feel less dizzy.

Patient (Man): What is that machine? What is it for?

Nurse(Woman): This is an incentive spirometer. It is to help you to breathe more deeply. Patients can get pneumonia after surgery because they are in pain and don't breathe deeply. This machine helps prevent pneumonia.

Patient (Man): Why did the doctor listen to my belly?

Nurse(Woman): He was listening for bowel sounds. As soon as your bowels are moving again, you can start to eat again.

Patient (Man): All I want to do is sleep. Why are you keeping me up?

Nurse (Woman): It is my job to make sure you don't have any complications. If you do the deep breathing and get out of bed often, you will be able to go home quicker.

Patient (Man): I'll try to do as you say.

This is the end of Part Three. Now look at Part Four.

You will hear a conversation between a nurse and a patient about the meals and food. Fill in the blanks. Write the answers on your answer sheet. You will hear the conversation twice.

Nurse (Woman): Welcome, Mr. Smith. I'm the nurse in charge of this ward. We hope you will feel at home here. This is Miss Rose Clinton.

Patient (Man): Sorry to bother you all.

Nurse (Woman): If you need anything, just press this button.

Patient (Man): Is it possible for my sister to stay here with me?

Nurse (Woman): Yes, but she has to pay for her bed. Does she want to have meals here too? We don't think it is necessary for her to stay. Your condition isn't so serious.

Patient (Man): What are the hours here for meals?

Nurse (Woman): Patients usually get up at 7 AM. Breakfast is at 8 AM. The ward rounds and treatments start at 9 AM. Lunch is at noon. After that it is nap time. Visiting hours are from 3 to 7 PM. Dinner is at 6 PM. Bed time is at 10 PM.

Patient (Man): Will you show me where the sitting-room, bathroom and telephone are?

Nurse (Woman): Of course. Here they are. Which kind of food do you prefer, Chinese or Western?

Patient (Man): I like Chinese food very much.

Nurse (Woman): Have you eaten breakfast already?

Patient (Man): Yes, I have.

Nurse (Woman): How is your appetite?

Patient (Man): Not so good.

Nurse (Woman): What are your eating habits?

Patient (Man): I don't eat much. I would like to have a snack in the afternoon and before going to bed.

Nurse (Woman): Are you allergic to any food?

Patient (Man): I am allergic to sea food.

Nurse (Woman): Do you like fruit?

Patient (Man): Yes, please give me some with each meal.

Nurse (Woman): Do you prefer porridge or a cream soup?

Patient (Man): I like rice porridge.

Nurse (Woman): Please try to eat a little more. It will help you recover more quickly.

This is the end of Part Four.

You now have five minutes to write your answers on the answer sheet.

You have one more minute.

This is the end of the listening test.

参考答案及解析

Ⅰ Listening

Part One

1. F　本题中病人自述头疼 headache，故选 F。
2. E　本题中病人自述腹痛，呕吐恶心，选项中只有阑尾炎符合这些症状，故选 E。
3. C　病人自述肺部疼痛，护士也提到肺部感染，故选 C。
4. A　护士提到给病人注射胰岛素，而且提醒病人要学会使用胰岛素笔，故选 A。
5. B　病人的血液检查显示血红蛋白偏低，可能是贫血症，故选 B。

Part Two

6. B　病人说她的疼痛有 3 hours，而不是题目中的 3 days，故本句错误。

7. B　根据对话，病人并没有 diarrhea 的症状，故本句错误。

8. A　根据对话，护士说病人有轻微发烧，故本句正确。

9. A　根据对话，护士说病人的 white blood cell count 是 $18 * 10^9$/L，故本句正确。

10. A　根据对话，护士说医生将会对病人实施手术，故本题正确。

Part Three

11. B　对话中护士说叫病人起床活动是为了 prevent complications，故选 B。

12. C　对话中护士说用诱发型肺量计是为了帮助病人呼吸，故选 C。

13. C　根据对话，使用这个机器可以帮助病人预防肺炎，故选 C。

14. A　根据对话，医生听病人的腹部是在听肠鸣音，故选 A。

15. A　根据对话，护士让病人起床活动从而避免并发症是他的工作职责，故选 A。

Part Four

16. 8/eight　根据护士的回答，早餐时间是早上 8 点。

17. 6/six　根据护士的回答，晚餐时间是晚上 6 点。

18. Chinese　病人的回答说他喜欢吃中餐。

19. sea　病人的回答说他对海鲜过敏。

20. porridge　病人的回答说，他喜欢喝大米粥。

Ⅱ　Reading and Writing

Part One

21. B　根据 B 段的叙述，Symptoms commonly include lower right abdominal pain，症状包括下腹部疼痛，可知题目描述的内容在此段有涉及。

22. D　根据 D 的叙述，贫血症的主要表现就是血红蛋白偏低。

23. C　根据 C 段描述，这种疾病是肺炎，哮喘是此段中描述的风险因素之一。

24. E　根据 E 的叙述，感染的过程是有一个发展的过程，并且最初可能不被注意到。

25. D　题干中提及的句子在 D 段中有很明显清楚的说明。

26. A　根据 A 中"The cough, however, may last for more than two weeks."可找到题干的出处。

27. F　题干中所说的血糖高以及尿频等症状就是 F 段中对此疾病症状的描述。

28. C　题干说 X 光胸片、血检、痰液培养分析可以帮助确诊，与 C 中"Chest X-ray, blood tests, and culture of the sputum may help confirm the diagnosis."相对应。

29. B　根据 B 段叙述"Symptoms commonly include lower right abdominal pain, nausea, vomiting, and decreased appetite."和题干意思是吻合的。

30. D　D 中对 anema 的描述，即"Anemia that comes on quickly often has greater symptoms, which may include confusion, feeling like one is going to pass out, loss of consciousness, or increased thirst."和题干意思一致。

Part Two

31. A　根据文章第一段，气味可以提供有关地点和人的信息，故正确。

32. B 根据第一段最后一句话的叙述，Randall Reed 是美国约翰霍普金斯大学研究嗅觉的专家，故错。

33. C 本文并没有讲到气味可以帮助警察侦查刑事案件，故本题选 C。

34. B 根据第二段的叙述，即使有一定距离，气味是能够给人们一些危险的警示的，故错误。

35. A 第二段的画线单词 alert 的意思是“警惕，警觉”，题目中的 on guard 也是“警觉”之意，故正确。

36. A 根据第二段最后一句描述，如果烤箱中有东西烧焦了，整个屋子的人都会知道。故正确。

37. B 根据第三段第一句话所述，“With just a simple scent, smell can also evoke very intense emotion.”仅仅是简单的气味，嗅觉就会引起强烈的情感，与题干中“It is impossible that smell can evoke very intense emotion.”嗅觉引起强烈的情感是不可能的意思相反，故本题错。

38. A 根据第三段中的描述，如果你的母亲在你 3 岁时就去世了，她曾经拥有一座花园，你不必去辨认那种气味或者有意识地回忆起你母亲或者她的花园，只要你闻到那种紫喇叭花的香味，你就会感到伤感。可知题干描述是正确的。

39. C 根据文章最后一段描述，人体的受体细胞很少，但并没有说明是否比动物的少，故本题应该选择“没有提及”这个答案。

40. A 根据文章最后一段的描述，无论是人还是动物，感知味道的主要因素取决于受体细胞，故本题正确。

Part Three

41. A 推理题，第一段第二句的意思是，我们中目前有三分之一的人患有过敏症，故而过敏症越来越普遍。

42. B 细节题，第二段第二句话“The immune system is there to protect the body against outside attackers, including viruses, bacteria and parasites.”提到免疫系统能够保护我们的身体免受外界物质的侵袭，这些物质包括病毒、细菌以及寄生虫。

43. C 推理题，第二段最后一句的意思是过敏者的免疫系统产生抗体是因为它们会错误地认定这些无害物质是危险的。

44. A 细节题，第三段第三句话提到，当一个人在多年正常食用坚果后，突然变得对其过敏，是因为其免疫系统在这一过程中认定坚果为危险物质并针对其产生了免疫抗体。

45. A 推理题，最后一段讲到肿胀 swelling 是过敏的一种症状，所以 B 选项正确，文章中反复提到过敏者体内的抗体在患者过敏的过程中是如何起作用的，所以 C 正确，A 选项说我们很安全是因为我们没有受到过敏物质的攻击，这一点文中并没有提及，所以本题答案选 A。

Part Four

46. C 首先医生需要检查并清洁伤口。

47. A 第二步是局部麻醉。

48. B 第三步是用针线缝合伤口。

49. F 第四步是给缝合线打结。

50. D　第五步是给伤口上敷料包扎伤口。

Part Five

51. D　填写本空应该根据词性前后一致的原则,句中连词 and 前是名词 blood,后面也应接一个名词,根据句意,"白血病涉及血液和造血器官",故填 organ。

52. F　本空填写应根据词性搭配,white blood cells 是名词,前面应该填一个形容词来修饰,根据句意,"患白血病的孩子会在骨碴中产生大量不正常的白细胞",故填 abnormal。

53. A　本空所在的分句仅有主语 white blood cells,而无谓语动词,故本空应填入一个动词的复数形式,以便与复数主语相配合。根据句意,唯有 fight 符合要求。

54. B　本空在介词 from 后面,应该填一个名词构成 protect ... from ... 的搭配。根据句意,"它们不能保护人体免受感染",故填 infections。

55. C　本空逗号后面的 infection-fighting 是一个分词短语作定语的结构,修饰 white blood cells,根据句意,"骨髓中不正常的白细胞的繁殖无法控制,使得骨髓中难以形成足够的正常抗感染的白细胞",唯有形容词 normal 符合要求。

56. G　本空在动词 carry 后面,应填一个名词从而构成动宾关系。根据句意,"红血细胞是将血液中的氧气运送到身体其他器官的细胞",唯有 oxygen 符合要求。

57. H　本空前是定冠词 the,后为名词短语,当然应填入形容词,根据句意,white 符合要求。

58. E　本空前为情态动词 may,故须填入一原形动词,根据句意,应选 move。

59. K　本空前为定冠词 the,且根据空前句意,应可判断此空为名词,为后 where 引导的定语从句的先行词,名词中唯 blood stream 符合要求。

60. I　此空前为系动词 is,可填入一形容词,且根据上下文,此处的句意是说白血病大多数情况下还是可以治愈的,故填 treatable。

Part Six

61.

A Care Plan Report

Mr. Jason Hoover, whose next of kin is his son, Leo Hoover, was admitted to the hospital with dehydration. The patient has such problems as inadequate fluid intake, dry and dehydrated skin, dry lips and coated tongue. His urinary output has also decreased. So the nursing goals include adequate hydration, moist lips and tongue, as well as a urinary output of at least 2,000 ml per day. And nursing interventions are as follows: ensure fluid at least 3,000 ml; sit the patient well before giving him drinks; offer drinks to the patient hourly (the patient prefers tea or lemon to coffee); give the patient mouth care every 4 hours; observe and record urinary output of the patient and report to the doctor if the output is still inadequate.

【审题】

本题要求写一份完整的护理计划。护理计划主要包括护理诊断或问题、护理目标和护理措施。本题中病人护理计划表所提供的信息比较齐全,所以只需将表中的单词或词组用适当的形式连成句子即可。写作中要注意信息的处理,不可遗漏任何重要信息,必要时可以重新组合,并使用适当的连词使前后句子语意连贯,重点突出。同时还需注意文体的规范性和句型的多样性，避免简单重复。

【范文评述】

本篇范文内容详实，涵盖了试题中提供的所有细节，包括病人的症状、问题及护理措施等。语言通顺，无病句或其他语法错误。在句型的使用方面也十分妥帖，如第一段用了非限定性定语从句，时态方面正确使用了过去时和完成时。此外，连词 so，and 等的使用让文章的逻辑性更清晰流畅。

医护英语水平考试(二级)

模拟训练(五)

听力文本

This is METS-2 Listening Test. There are four parts in the test, Parts One, Two, Three, and Four. You will hear each part twice. Now, look at the instructions for Part One.

You will hear five patients describing their problems. Decide what problem each patient has. Write the appropriate letter A-H in each box. Mark the corresponding letter on your answer sheet. You will hear each conversation twice.

Here is an example:

Nurse (Woman): Good morning. What's wrong with you?

Patient (Man): I have a severe pain in my joints for more than one week.

Nurse (Woman): Does it become sharper in rainy days?

Patient (Man): Yes, that's right.

The answer is arthritis, so write letter E in the box.

Now we are ready to start.

Conversation 1

Nurse (Woman): Good morning. What seems to be the trouble?

Patient (Man): Several days ago, my chest felt tight and I even couldn't breathe at that moment.

Nurse (Woman): How often does it happen these days?

Patient (Man): Every two or three days.

Conversation 2

Nurse (Woman): Good morning, Mr. White. How are you today?

Patient (Man): Nice to see you again. I'm fine, thanks.

Nurse (Woman): Great. I need to check your blood glucose level before you see the doctor. Is that OK?
Patient (Man): Yes, that's fine with me.
Nurse (Woman): Let's wait for the result to flash on the screen. Oh, still 8, but it is lower than yesterday.

Conversation 3

Nurse (Woman): Have you got better now?
Patient (Man): No, awful, my back still hurts a lot.
Nurse (Woman): Don't worry, the doctor will come soon.
Patient (Man): Thanks, it's really annoyed me a lot.

Conversation 4

Nurse (Woman): Hello, Mr. Green. I've got your lunch as well as some new things to help you feed yourself.
Patient (Man): Oh, yes?
Nurse (Woman): Since you started on a thickened liquid diet yesterday, the OT's sent you a non-slip bowl and this modified utensil. It's easy for you to hold.
Patient (Man): Right, well, I'll try them out.

Conversation 5

Nurse (Woman): You look pale, Mr. Simpson. What's your problem?
Patient (Man): I often feel tired these days.
Nurse (Woman): Oh really? I'm sorry to hear that. Any other symptom?
Patient (Man): I don't want to eat anything either.
Nurse (Woman): I suppose you are under much pressure recently.

This is the end of Part One. Now look at Part Two.
You will hear a conversation between a patient and a nurse about the test results. For each of the following sentences, decide whether it is True (A) or False (B). Put a tick (√) in the relevant box. Mark the corresponding letter on your answer sheet. You will hear the conversation twice.
Nurse (Man): Good morning, are you Amelia?
Patient (Woman): Good morning, Nurse. Yes, I am.
Nurse (Man): Nice to meet you. Take a seat, please.
Patient (Woman): OK, thank you.
Nurse (Man): Are you still feeling nauseous at the moment?
Patient (Woman): No, I haven't felt sick since I finished my ultrasound test.
Nurse (Man): Great. By the way, your test results came in just now.

Patient (Woman): What do they say? Are they good news or bad?

Nurse (Man): Your temperature, pulse, blood pressure and weight are normal. Erm ... that's really good.

Patient (Woman): Yes, sounds great. What about ultrasound?

Nurse (Man): After the ultrasound, it looks like the fetal heart sound is clear and within normal limits.

Patient (Woman): I'm glad to hear that.

Nurse (Man): But here, it showed the position of the fetus is a bit too low.

Patient (Woman): Gosh! I was afraid you were going to say that!

Nurse (Man): Don't get too worried! We still need to get to the bottom of this and tell you what to do.

Patient (Woman): Wow, that's a load off my mind. Thank you.

Nurse (Man): Thanks for your cooperation.

This is the end of Part Two. Now look at Part Three.

You will hear a conversation between a patient and a nurse about pain. For each of the following questions or unfinished sentences, choose the correct answer A, B or C. Put a tick (√) in the relevant box. Mark the corresponding letter on your answer sheet. You will hear the conversation twice.

Nurse(Woman): Hello, Mr. Jameson. How are you feeling today?

Patient (Man): Hello, Judy! I feel a bit down today. I've got a lot of pain.

Nurse (Woman): Oh, I'm sorry to hear that. I've got a pain chart so you can explain your pain a bit better.

Patient (Man): All right. There are two areas which hurt.

Nurse (Woman): OK. Can you show me the first one of your body?

Patient (Man): It's around my prostate.

Nurse (Woman): Mm, it's where the main cancer is, isn't it? What's the pain like?

Patient (Man): Yes. It's an aching pain.

Nurse (Woman): I see. Can you describe your pain on a scale of zero to ten?

Patient (Man): Maybe around six. And it turns worse when I get out of the bed to walk around.

Nurse (Woman): OK, I see. What do you take for the pain?

Patient (Man): A syringe driver with morphine makes it better.

Nurse (Woman): OK, what about the next pain?

Patient (Man): On my left arm, and it is an infected wound.

Nurse (Woman): How do you describe this pain?

Patient (Man): It's around two. But the wound is aching especially when the dressing is changed.

Nurse (Woman): Got it. I should get you some painkillers before the dressing change and a non-stick dressing will make the pain better.

Patient(Man): Thank you very much.

Nurse (Woman): Would you like a cup of tea, too?

Patient (Man): Great, Judy, I'd like that.

This is the end of Part Three. Now look at Part Four.

You will hear a conversation between a doctor and a patient about the discharge medication. Fill in the blanks. Write the answers on your answer sheet. You will hear the conversation twice.

Doctor (Woman): Good morning. This is your discharge medication list. Shall I have a check?

Patient (Man): OK.

Doctor (Woman): What's your name, please?

Patient (Man): John Feldman, and I'm 42.

Doctor (Woman): That's right. I've got the medication from the pharmacy, Mr. Feldman. I just need to explain a few things to you.

Patient (Man): Oh good. I was waiting for that.

Doctor (Woman): This capsule is your antibiotic. Make sure you take it on an empty stomach and twice a day.

Patient (Man): Oh right. Take it before eating.

Doctor (Woman): The second is your eye drops. They last only a month so remember to discard the contents after this date.

Patient (Man): OK. Before November 23rd. I got it.

Doctor (Woman): Do you know where the suitable place is to keep eye drops?

Patient (Man): As far as I can see, I must avoid too much sun with them, so they should be kept in the fridge.

Doctor (Woman): Good. The last one is the lotion for your rash.

Patient (Man): What should I pay attention to?

Doctor (Woman): It's important that you shake the bottle so you can mix the contents well.

Patient (Man): Oh yes. Thanks for reminding me.

Doctor (Woman): That's all right.

This is the end of Part Four.

You now have five minutes to write your answers on the answer sheet. You have one more minute. This is the end of the listening test.

参考答案及解析

Ⅰ Listening

Part One

1. D　本题中病人自述胸闷，呼吸不畅(my chest felt tight and I even couldn't breathe at that moment)，故选 D 哮喘。

2. G　本题中护士给病人检查血糖值，故选 G 糖尿病。

3. F　病人自述背疼，故选 F。

4. C　病人需进流食，言语治疗师让他使用防滑碗和改良器皿帮助自主进食，说明病人吞咽困难，故选 C。

5. B　病人自述乏力，不想吃东西，故选 B 没有胃口。

Part Two

6. B　女士说做完超声波检查之后没有恶心的反应，故本句错误。

7. A　根据对话，病人做了一个超声波检查，故本句正确。

8. B　根据对话，检查结果基本不错，但是胎儿位置有点偏低，故本句错误。

9. B　根据对话，当女士听说胎儿位置偏低时有点害怕，故本句错误。

10. A　对话中提及呕吐、胎儿及各项检查，故可认为这位女士在做产前检查，故本句正确。

Part Three

11. A　病人的第一处疼痛位于前列腺周围，故选 A。

12. C　第一处疼痛是因为病人的主要病因——前列腺癌，故选 C。

13. C　根据对话，病人认为使用注射器泵能缓减第一处疼痛，故选 C。

14. B　根据对话，病人自评第二处疼痛为二级，故选 B。

15. B　根据对话，换敷料的时候第二处疼痛尤为明显，故选 B。

Part Four

16. 42　根据病人的回答来确定。

17. antibiotic　第一种药是抗生素胶囊。

18. twice　抗生素空腹服用，一天两次。

19. discard　滴眼液在有效期之后必须弃用。

20. shake　皮疹洗液，用前摇匀。

Ⅱ Reading and Writing

Part One

21. B　B 段中提到，When a kidney is removed from a living donor, it is not necessary to use elaborate preservation techniques. 肾脏从捐赠者身上移植后不一定必须使用精密的技术保存。因为后文说到捐体的摘除手术和受体的移植手术是同时进行的。

22. D　D 段提到 For a kidney to be preserved from 48 to 72 hours, a complicated

machine is required to provide artificial circulation. 肾脏要保存 48 到 72 小时就需要复杂的机器提供人工循环,说明仅用低温保存就不够了,据此可判断题干的出处。

23. F 根据“these fluids have damaging effects”说明对肾脏等器官有不好的影响。

24. B B段中提到,The operations on the donor and receiver are performed at the same time,取出和接受肾脏的手术可以同时进行,即取出后马上移植到受者体内,据此可判断题干的出处。

25. E E段中说到:血细胞、精子和某些游离的组织细胞可以在零度以下存活,此即 25 题的依据。

26. C 根据C中“Cool solutions are put into the blood vessels of the kidney, which is then kept at 4℃ in a refrigerator or surrounded by ice in a vacuum bottle”在肾脏血管中注入冷却液体,放在 4℃的冰箱或在真空瓶中用冰块保存。

27. A 根据A中叙述,大脑若无血液供给,在 3~5 分钟之内就会死亡,据此可判断题干的出处。

28. C 题干说肾脏需要保存在真空中,与C中“surrounded by ice in a vacuum bottle”相对应。

29. D D段中提到 To keep a kidney undamaged for longer than 72 hours is difficult. 据此可判断题干的出处。

30. A A段中提到 the cornea can be removed for grafting at relative leisure. 角膜移植可以相对来说从容一些,据此可判断题干的出处。

Part Two

31. A 根据文章第一段第一句话,科学家将死亡分为临床死亡和生物死亡两种类型,故正确。

32. B 根据第一段末句的叙述,生物死亡应该指生物体的改变对细胞和组织造成永久性损坏,不是心脏暂停跳动,故错误。

33. A 根据全文大意和文章题目,本文主要叙述科学家在寻求延长临床死亡的方法,故本题正确。

34 B 根据第三段的叙述,冷却应该是延缓对身体组织的破坏,而非“speed up”加速,意思相反,故错误。

35. C 题干说“年轻雌狒狒是最佳实验对象”,但文章中并未提到最佳实验对象的物种、性别和年龄。

36. A 根据第三段叙述,给 Keta 用麻醉药后开始实验,narcotic 与 anaesthetic 都是麻醉剂。

37. B 根据第三段“The monkey's blood pressure decreased and an hour later both the heart and respiration stopped”狒狒的血压下降,一小时后心脏和呼吸停止,与题干中“blood pressure became higher”相反,故本题错。

38. B 根据第三段中“After fifteen minutes, spontaneous respiration began.”十五分钟后开始自主呼吸,可知题干中“立即有呼吸”错误。

39. A 根据文章的最后三句话:“两分钟后,狒狒的心脏开始跳动。15 分钟后,自主呼吸恢复;四小时后,她睁开眼睛。她的行为和健康动物几乎没有任何区别。”说明实验结束后狒狒恢复了健康，故本题正确。

40. A 本题是推测题，科学家做此实验后，找到了使心脏再次工作的方法，其目的在于降低心脏病的致命率，故正确。

Part Three

41. B 推理题，第一段第一句告诉我们由于DNA是可遗传的，因此同一个家庭、部落甚至种族的人们可能会(因为共同的祖先)而拥有相同的DNA链。

42. C 细节题，第一段第二句提到宗谱学可以帮助DNA这种遗传标记独一无二的特性来推断一个人与家族中其他人的关系。

43. A 推理题，第二段第三句告诉我们一旦分子宗谱学研究小组所建立的数据库收集了充足的全世界遗传结构样本，他们将能够解决以前单纯依靠传统史料所不能解决的宗谱问题。

44. B 推理题，第三段第二句话提到如果有两个姓氏相同的人怀疑他们有血缘关系，但又没有书面材料加以证明，我们就分析他们的DNA采样，寻找共同的遗传标记。

45. C 推理题，第一段第三句告诉我们以遗传标记，即DNA分析为手段的宗谱学可以克服因领养、私生或者记录缺失等原因造成的家族信息不全问题，因此C不正确。

Part Four

46. B 使用起吊装置的第一步是向病人解释该装置的重要性。

47. A 第三步是让病人抬起手臂，把吊带系到起吊装置上。

48. E 第五步是将病人扶起，变成站姿。

49. F 第七步是让病人先尝试走几步。

50. C 第八步是让病人连续走一小会儿。

Part Five

51. B 减肥即节食之意，go on diets。

52. H 本空后为and，连词连接前后两个相等的部分，根据and之后的sugars推断本空需要填入一个名词，再结合句意，节食的关键是要少摄入脂肪和糖分，故选fats。

53. A 本空前有连词or，连接前后相等部分，前面都是动宾搭配结构，据此推断本空也是动宾搭配，需要填一个名词。结合句意，其他减肥的办法还有使用仪器、服用药物和动手术，故选surgery。

54. L being后接形容词构成系表结构，结合句意，对大多数人来说，身材好意味着瘦，故选thin。

55. F 本空前有worry about，说明后面要填一个名词构成动宾搭配。再根据后面一句Many doctors say being overweight is not healthy. 说明很多人担心自己的健康，故选health。

56. D 本空后有名词country，需要一个形容词修饰。再根据第三段的数据，可判断出美国是世界上超重人口最多的国家，选overweight。

57. G 本空前为定冠词the，后为名词fat，这种情况多半要求填入一个形容词修饰fat。所给选项中C、G、L都为形容词，根据句子意思，唯有G选项的stored符合要求。

58. C 本空后有and，连词连接前后两个相等的部分，根据and后的easy判断本空需要一个形容词，再结合句意，快速简单的减肥方法，故选fast。

59. J 本空是动词和副词搭配,减掉脂肪 take off fat。

60. I 根据句子结构,判断本句缺少谓语动词,再结合句意,每本书都承诺可以减肥,故选 promises。

Part Six

61.

A Patient Admission Report

Jasmine Miller is a 74-year-old lady who was admitted to the hospital on Sep. 15, 2017. She complained that her blood pressure was higher than normal for more than one week and often felt dizzy these days.

Signs and symptoms of the patient include: frequent urination, increased thirst and hunger, dizziness and fatigue. Diagnosis shows that the patient has diabetes.

Major nursing instructions for the patient are as follows: a) The patient should inject insulin three times a day. b) Medications for diabetes and hypertension are necessary for the patient. c) The patient needs to keep healthy diets in daily life to control sugar strictly.

【审题】

这是一篇关于病人入院报告的写作。要求考生写 100 词以上,内容应包括:病人姓名、年龄、入院时间、症状、诊断、医嘱等。表格中的主要信息要表述完整,无遗漏;但也要注意不要超词太多。考生应注意使用常见的表达用语,如:be admitted to the hospital /be hospitalized; signs and symptoms of the patient include ... ; as follows 等。

【范文评述】

本篇范文内容详实,涵盖了试题中提供的主要信息,包括病人的症状、诊断及医嘱等。语言通顺,无语法错误,时态的使用亦较为妥帖,如第一段主要用过去时,因陈述过去的事实,如入院时间、主诉等;而第二、三两段则主要使用一般现在时,因其内容为病人症状及医嘱。在语言使用上也有可圈可点之处,如:第二段的 include 后的宾语均为名词性短语,而第三段的注意事项则均用完整的句子表达。

医护英语水平考试(二级)

模拟训练(六)

听力文本

This is METS-2 Listening Test. There are four parts in the test, Parts One, Two, Three, and Four. You will hear each part twice. Now, look at the instructions for Part One.

You will hear five patients describing their problems. Decide what problem each patient

has. Write the appropriate letter A-H in each box. Mark the corresponding letter on your answer sheet. You will hear each conversation twice.
Here is an example:
Nurse (Woman): Good morning. What seems to be your problem?
Patient (Man): I've had a terrible headache for the last two days.
Nurse (Woman): Did you vomit?
Patient (Man): No, I didn't.
The answer is headache, so write letter E in the box. Now we are ready to start.

Conversation 1

Nurse (Woman): Good morning. What seems to be the trouble?
Patient (Man): I don't feel very well. Perhaps I've got heat-stroke.
Nurse (Woman): Can I take your temperature?
Patient (Man): Sure.

Conversation 2

Nurse (Woman): Have you tried the throat spray, Mr. Black?
Patient (Man): Yes, and I'm feeling much relieved now.
Nurse (Woman): Continue to use it for another three days.
Patient (Man): Still three times a day?
Nurse (Woman): Yes, you will feel OK again.

Conversation 3

Nurse (Woman): Good morning. What seems to be the trouble?
Patient (Man): I can't sleep well recently, and I find it difficult to fall asleep.
Nurse (Woman): How long have you had this problem?
Patient (Man): For one month.
Nurse (Woman): Let me take your blood pressure.

Conversation 4

Nurse (Woman): Which department do you want to register with?
Patient (Man): I don't know which clinic. I have a rash all over my body. It aches badly.
Nurse (Woman): I think you should see a dermatologist first. If necessary we'll transfer you to the physician.
Patient (Man): OK. Thank you very much.

Conversation 5

Nurse (Woman): What brings you to the emergency room? Where don't you feel well?
Patient (Man): Nurse, I suddenly developed a sharp pain in my upper abdomen.

Nurse (Woman): What kind of pain is it? Intermittent or persistent?
Patient (Man): It's a kind of sharp pain. It was off and on, but now it's all the time.

This is the end of Part One. Now look at Part Two.
You will hear a conversation between a patient and a doctor about diarrhea. For each of the following sentences, decide whether it is True (A) or False (B). Put a tick (√) in the relevant box. Mark the corresponding letter on your answer sheet. You will hear the conversation twice.
Doctor (Woman): Mr. Johnson, when did your diarrhea start?
Patient (Man): It started last night.
Doctor (Woman): Do you remember how many times you went to the toilet?
Patient (Man): I can't remember exactly. It must have been over 10 times.
Doctor (Woman): What kind of stool did you notice, watery or mucous?
Patient (Man): At first it was watery, but it is mucous now.
Doctor (Woman): Do you feel abdominal pain when you go to the toilet?
Patient (Man): Yes.
Doctor (Woman): Have you vomited?
Patient (Man): No, but I feel nauseated.
Doctor(Woman): I'll take a sample of your stool for examination. Your condition doesn't seem serious, but we must give you intravenous infusion to prevent dehydration and antibiotics as well.
Patient (Man): Thank you.

This is the end of Part Two. Now look at Part Three.
You will hear a conversation between a patient and a doctor about heartburn. For each of the following questions or unfinished sentences, choose the correct answer A, B or C. Put a tick (√) in the relevant box. Mark the corresponding letter on your answer sheet. You will hear the conversation twice.
Doctor (Woman): Good morning, Mr. Wilson. What can I do for you this morning?
Patient (Man): Good morning, Doctor. Same old thing—heartburn. It seems to be getting worse. I'm sick of it.
Doctor (Woman): Let me just have a look at your notes. I see you've been coming to us once a month for some time. Let me ask you a few questions, just to see if we've missed something, or to see if you've left anything out.
Patient (Man): All right. What do you want to know?
Doctor (Woman): Well, when did you first have this problem? How long is it since you noticed it seemed to be getting worse? And do you understand about heartburn?
Patient (Man): It must have been about eighteen months ago when I first noticed it. It was a rush of stomach acid up into my mouth. That's heartburn, isn't it? It seems to have

got worse last fortnight.

Doctor (Woman): Yes. When have you been getting it? Usually before meals? Or after meals? And have you noticed any particular kind of other discomfort or pain, perhaps associated with the heartburn?

Patient (Man): Generally, after. I haven't felt any other special pain anywhere with it, no.

Doctor (Woman): When you say "after meals"—is that long after? Or shortly after?

Patient (Man): Usually shortly after. I do a kind of burp—and then this acid shoots up into my mouth. Very unpleasant.

Doctor (Woman): I know—I get a slight burp occasionally myself—but only when I've had too much to eat. You know, made a bit of a pig of myself. Mine's not a chronic condition, like yours seems to be. But you're not regularly over-eating, are you?

Doctor (Man): No, I'm not. I never, in fact.

This is the end of Part Three. Now look at Part Four.

You will hear a conversation between a doctor and a patient about the treatment of fracture. Fill in the blanks. Write the answers on your answer sheet. You will hear the conversation twice.

Doctor (Woman): What seems to be the problem?

Patient (Man): Well, I was crossing the road, where a car came round the corner too quickly, and when the driver saw me, it was too late to stop. I was knocked to the ground, and when I got up, my left arm and elbow were grazed and now, I have a pain in my ribs.

Doctor (Woman): I'll just take a look. Where does it hurt?

Patient (Man): It's hard to say. It hurts all over.

Doctor (Woman): Does it hurt when I do this?

Patient (Man): Ouch! The pain is very bad when you press here.

Doctor (Woman): Your arm and elbow seem to be all right. But, to be on the safe side, you'd better go to the X-ray Department. When the X-rays are ready, bring them back to me.

Patient (Man): OK. See you later.

Doctor (Woman): See you then!

(Ten minutes later, the patient brings back the X-ray plates.)

Patient (Man): Doctor, here's my X-rays.

Doctor (Woman): I'll just take a look at it. Everything is all right, except here, see it? There's a hairline fracture?

Patient (Man): Is it serious?

Doctor (Woman): No. It's not very serious, but you should take two or three weeks off work, and rest in bed as much as possible.

Patient (Man): Should I take some medicine, Doctor?
Doctor (Woman): All right. I'll give you some herbal medicine to help you heal quickly. In addition, I will prescribe you some medicine for oral administration. Here is a prescription. Take it to the chemist's. Please take the medicine according to the instruction.
Patient (Man): Will I need to be put in plaster?
Doctor (Woman): No, it isn't necessary. I have prescribed you a tube of ointment. Administer it two or three times a day.
Patient (Man): Thank you very much, Doctor.
Doctor (Woman): Not at all. Goodbye!
Patient (Man): Goodbye!

This is the end of Part Four. You now have five minutes to write your answers on the answer sheet. You have one more minute. This is the end of the listening test.

参考答案及解析

Ⅰ Listening

Part One

1. H 病人自述中暑(heat-stroke),故选 H。

2. B 本题一开始护士问病人有没有试过用咽喉喷雾(throat spray),由此推断病人的问题是咽喉问题,故选 B(咽喉炎)。

3. G 病人自述睡不好,很难入睡,故选 G(失眠)。

4. A 病人自述皮疹(rash),故选 A。

5. F 病人出现上腹部疼痛,选项中只有 F(胃痛)符合,故选 F。

Part Two

6. A 医生问病人去了多少次厕所,病人回答"一定有 10 次以上",故本句正确。

7. B 病人起先是有水样便,然后现在才出现有粘液,故本句说病人的大便一直都有粘液,不正确。

8. B 医生问病人有没有呕吐,病人说没有呕吐,只有恶心的感觉,故本句说病人呕吐了好几个小时,不正确。

9. A 医生告诉病人需要取大便做检查,故本句正确。

10. B 对话中医生说要给病人静脉滴注(infusion)而不是静脉推注(injection),故本句错误。

Part Three

11. A 根据病人的理解,heartburn(胃灼热)是胃酸涌到口腔里,故 A 选项正确。heartburn 与心脏无关,C 不正确;病人出现胃灼热主要是饭后,故 B 选项也不正确。

12. B 病人自诉病症在 fortnight(两星期)前变得更糟,故选 B。

13. B　病人在回答医生提问病症出现的具体时间时提到是 shortly after meals(饭后不久),故选 B。

14. A　病人描述胃灼痛出现时的症状,用 very unpleasant(很难受),故选 A。

15. C　医生提到自己也有打嗝的问题,主要出现在吃过多的时候,为的是提醒病人不要吃太多,故 A 选项(建议病人多吃)不正确;而 B 选项博得病人的同情也不合适;故选 C,安抚病人的情绪。

Part Four

16. knocked　病人被车撞倒在地。

17. ribs　病人陈述左手手臂和手肘擦伤,而且肋骨部位疼痛。

18. X-ray　医生建议病人去放射科做 X 光检查。

19. fracture　根据 X 光检查结果,医生诊断病人有骨裂(hairline fracture)。

20. herbal　对于病人的治疗,医生开了一些中草药(herbal)、口服西药及一管药膏。

Ⅱ　Reading and Writing

Part One

21. D　根据题干中的 food marketing and poor policymaking 可以定位到 D 段的最后一句:"Researchers say the world's obesity problem is a result of food marketing and poor policymaking in many areas."

22. A　题干定义肥胖为身体里有大量的脂肪,与原文 A 段中"Obesity is a condition in which the body stores large, unhealthy amounts of fat."的描述一致。

23. E　题干中"so expensive that poor people can't afford"(如此贵以至于穷人都负担不起),在 E 段中能找到相同意义的句子"being priced out of reach, and especially out of reach of poor"(它的价格超出了穷人的承受范围),句型不同,语义完全相同。

24. D　根据题干中"the growth of childhood obesity has slowed"大致定位到 D 段中的句子"In countries where wages are higher, the growth of childhood obesity has slowed, but remains high."与题干中的句子比较,两句只是语序上的不同,基本属于原句复现的情况。

25. D　基于题干中的时间状语"a few decades ago",可以大致定位到 D 段,原文中"a few decades ago, there may have been very little obesity"表达有很少肥胖的情况,与题干中的描述"你几乎看不到很多肥胖的孩子",意义相同。

26. B　用具体的数字定位是比较简单的方法,如果篇章中没有其他相同的数字,基本可以快速找准答案,此题目即可用 130 million 快速找到 B 段中的描述。

27. F　该题干很短,只有一个新信息点"cancers",而原文 F 段中"Being overweight can cause many diseases later in life, including heart disease, stroke, diabetes and some cancers."有 cancers 一词,两个句子的语义也相同。

28. C　从题干中的"east Asia"可以大致定位到 C 段中的句子"... Middle Income Countries in areas such as East Asia ...",符合题干的意思"东亚属于中等收入国家"。

29. F　本题中有两处单词替换:题干中的'school performance'在 F 段中用"educational performance";题干中的'is influenced by'在 F 段中用'has a big effect on',表

达不同,语义相同。

30. B 在原文中提及 Body Mass Index(BMI 身体质量指数)只有 B 段,结合该短语上一句的描述“The researchers examined height and weight data for about 130 million people. They used this information to get the Body Mass Index measurements of the subjects.”可知 BMI 是与身高体重相关的。

Part Two

31. A 根据原文第一段“... we overuse some muscles. And that overuse can lead to strain and injury”,与题干句子表达一致,故此句正确。

32. B 题干句子意思为“使用电子产品的人经常耸肩膀(shrug their shoulders)”,但原文第二段中的句子“Many people who use tech devices also hunch their shoulders forward.”(很多使用电子产品的人经常向前隆起肩膀)。这两个动作是不一样的,所以本句错误。

33. A 原文第三段开头“constantly looking down at our devices creates an unnatural curve in our spine. This can cause nerve pain and other problems.”(不停地低头看电子产品使我们的脊柱不自然弯曲,这样的弯曲会引起神经痛和其他问题。)与本题题干意思一致,故正确。

34. C 该句题干意思为“看太多电视对颈部有害。”原文中所讲内容都针对“hand-held technology”(拿在手上的电子设备),跟看电视无关,故选 C。

35. A 原文中第三段结尾句“... it causes nerve pain and herniation(s) and different muscle tension headaches—different things that really can reduce quality of life.”中提及神经痛和紧张性头痛可能会降低生活质量,符合题干意思,故正确。

36. A 原文第四段开头“Common symptoms of tech neck are neck pain, loss of feeling in your hands and fingers, headaches ...”讲常见症状中有包括头痛,故此题正确。

37. B 原文第四段讲症状时描述为“In the worst cases of tech neck, you can lose the strength in your hands and fingers.”失去的是手和手指的力量,而不是如该题题干中描述的失去手指,故此题错误。

38. A 该句题干意思为“Fielding 女士的课帮助有颈椎病(科技颈)的人”,与原文中第四段的句子“she created a class to directly address the problem of tech neck.”意思一致,故此题正确。

39. C 题干的意思是:“将电话拿到跟眼睛水平的位置,可以舒缓上身的紧张。”这在原文第五段讲改善颈椎病的方法中未提及,故选择 C 答案。

40. B 原文第五段讲改善颈椎病的方法中,提及“Move your eyes to the screen, not your neck, head or shoulders.”(移动眼睛,而不是移动脖子、头或者肩膀。)这与题干意思相悖,故此题错误。

Part Three

41. A 在医学文章中经常出现一些专业词汇,对专业词汇的解析有很多种方法,该文章中用破折号解析的方式即是其中一种常用的方法,因此对破折号后面句子的理解就是本题的关键。probiotics(益生菌)的意思是“so-called ‘good’ bacteria that aid in digestion”(它是一种所谓的“好的”细菌,有助于消化),故该题选择 A 答案,beneficial 意为“有益的”;

microbe 意为细菌或微生物。

42. B　定位到文章第二段的句子"There are about 300 to 500 bacterial species that live in the human gut. Many help with digestion and keep the gastrointestinal system working right."其中讲到益生菌"help with digestion",故A选项正确;益生菌"live in the human gut",故C选项正确;与B选项相关的句子在第一段结尾"help to lessen symptoms of depression",益生菌可以帮助减轻抑郁的症状,而不是B选项中所描述的"can help cure depression"能帮助治愈抑郁症。故不正确的描述应该选B。

43. A　根据题干"New evidence shows"定位到原文第三段第二句话"there is also new evidence that shows probiotics can also affect a person's mental state, or mood",句中的affect在选项A中被have an effect on替换,故选择A。

44. C　对IBS(肠道易激综合征)的症状描述可以定位到原文第四段"Bercik notes that between 40 and 90 percent of people with irritable bowel syndrome, or IBS, also suffer from symptoms of anxiety and depression"和第五段"It causes stomach pains and can interfere with the body's waste removal process",故选项C未提到。

45. C　根据原文第四段中的句子"Bercik notes that between 40 and 90 percent of people with irritable bowel syndrome",作为加拿大的研究者Bercik,他研究40%～90%的IBS加拿大患者,与A选项的"超过一半的人"不一致,故A不正确。根据原文第六段第一句话"What we found was that the patients who were treated with this probiotic bacterium improved their gut's symptoms, but also surprisingly decreased their depression scores. That means their mood improved."(我们发现,用益生菌治疗的病人,不仅他们的肠道方面的症状得以改善,而且令人惊奇的是他们的抑郁评分分数下降,意味着情绪得以改善。)这与选项C的描述一致。而定位到原文第七段第一句话,Bercik说还需要做更大型的研究来确认这个结果,即有心理疾病的病人是否可以用益生菌来治疗还不能下定论,所以选项B也不正确,最终选择答案C。

Part Four

46. E　做核磁共振的第一步是身体和心理上的准备,根据第二步的后一句话提示"你被推进到扫描仪是头先进去还是脚先进去,依赖于你要扫描的身体部位。"由此推断前一句话应该是还未被推进到扫描仪,故答案E说"在被推进扫描仪前你要躺在平的床上"刚好前后逻辑一致。

47. C　根据第三步的前一句,我们了解这一步讲的是核磁共振的操作者,故接上文继续讲放射科医师如何操控机器。答案选C,但选项应该使用"He controls ... "会更好的接上文的单数名词。

48. B　上一个步骤提到放射科医师radiographer,B选项中的"the radiographer"刚好承接,句子内容也接得上,故选B。

49. A　根据第五步前一句的描述,提到扫描仪会发出噪音,作为处理办法,选择A"戴上耳塞或耳机",符合逻辑前后关系。

50. D　第六步的后半句提到扫描时间可能是15到90分钟,而前一句的选择只需在选项D和F中判断,F的内容与前面的第四步重复,故不合适,D选项表示"全程需要保持安静不动(虽然时间可能会比较长)",前后可以承接上。

Part Five

51. F　此空前的谓语动词搭配为“help (to) do ... ”故该空需要填动词原形,选项 F 为动词原形,填在此处表示“维生素 D 帮助身体吸收钙。”语意正确。

52. H　此空位于不定冠词 a 后面,应该是一个名词。该句子前面讲维生素 D 帮助身体吸收钙,从下文推断,它在神经、肌肉和免疫系统也有一定的作用,“have a role in ... ”(在……方面起到一定的作用),故答案 H 合适。

53. K　此空前提到人体获得钙的三种途径,“through your skin, from your diet, and from ... ”,所以需要填名词,又符合意思的只有 K(维生素 D 补充剂)。

54. C　此空属固定搭配,“exposure to ... ”(暴露于),整句的意思为“晒太阳后,你的身体自然而然会产生维生素 D”。

55. A　此空需要名词,和 bone 连在一起构成“bone density”(骨密度),缺乏维生素 D 会导致骨密度损失。

56. L　接上一句骨密度损失,跟一个定语从句,解释骨密度损失的危害,它会引起骨质疏松和骨折。contribute to 引起,促成,符合语义,故选 L。

57. D　该句提到佝偻病引起骨头变软以及________,此空有两个选择:其一,and 并列两个形容词“soft and ________”;其二,and 并列两个动词“become soft and ________”。所以暂定选项 B 和 D,语义也都符合,由于每个选项只能用一次,下文需要 B,故此空选择 D。

58. B　此空需要形容词修饰 bones,根据上下文的意思,故只有 B 适合。

59. E　此空也是需要形容词修饰后面的名词 connections,剩下一个 E 选项是形容词,故选 E,放到句子中,“研究人员正在研究维生素 D 与一些疾病的可能联系”,语义正确。

60. J　此空需要名词,又因为有“the effect ... on ... ”(对……的作用),故选 J。

Part Six

61.

A Case Report

John Brown, a 56-year-old male, was admitted to the hospital on July 7, 2017. He complained that he has had a bad cough, chest pain and shortness of breath for over two weeks.

Signs and symptoms of the patient include: a temperature of 37.8℃, severe cough, productive yellow and greenish sputum and difficulty breathing. The patient was diagnosed with chronic bronchitis.

Major nursing instructions for him are as follows: a) Have a good rest and drink much water. b) Do not have spicy food. c) Do not smoke or drink alcohol. d) Use some cough medicine and antibiotics if necessary.

【审题】

这是一篇病人入院登记表,也是二级作文常考的表格题型。表格中的信息常包括:病人基本信息(姓名、年龄、性别、出生日期、职业等)、入院日期及原因或主述、症状及检查结果(包括生命体征)、诊断和护理指导。学会使用和掌握一些常用的表达句型可以达到以不变应万变的效果,如下图所示:

表格中的表述	常用句型
Chief Complaint/Problem/Reason for Admission	Pt. complained of/that ... /Pt. was admitted ... with ...
Physical Exam/Signs and Symptoms	The examination showed that ... /On examination, Pt. ... /Signs and symptoms include ...
Diagnosis	Pt. was diagnosed with ...
Needs/Point to note/Instructions	Pt. should ... /needs to ... /... instructions include/are as follows:...

二级作文要求100个词，应将表格里的主要信息描述清楚，不要任意添加无关内容。行文时还要注意时态的选择。病人基本信息一般多使用一般现在时；入院情况多为一般过去式；症状和检查结果以及诊断通常用一般过去式；而护理指导是对病人的指导意见，常用一般现在时。

【范文评述】

本篇范文内容完整，涵盖了试题中提供的所有信息。语言通顺，恰当使用了固定句型结构，如"... was admitted ... complained that ... was diagnosed with ... 等"。无病句或其他语法错误。在时态的使用方面也十分妥帖，能根据描述内容变换使用恰当的时态，而不是一味使用某种固定的时态。范文将表格内容分成三个部分，思路清晰，一目了然，在语言使用上也有较多变化。

医护英语水平考试（二级）

模拟训练（七）

听力文本

This is METS-2 Listening Test. There are four parts in the test, Parts One, Two, Three, and Four. You will hear each part twice. Now, look at the instructions for Part One.

You will hear patients describing their pains. Decide what kind of pain each patient has. Write the appropriate letter A-H in each box. Mark the corresponding letter on your answer sheet. You will hear each conversation twice.

Here is an example:

Nurse (Woman): Mr. Heath, does your knee hurt?

Patient (Man): Yes, nurse, it does hurt and feels numb.

Nurse (Woman): Let me have a look first.
Patient (Man): Yes, please.
The answer is numbness, so write letter F in the box. Now we are ready to start.

Conversation 1

Nurse (Woman): Hello, Mr. Adams. Can you tell me what the problem is?
Patient (Man): I have an ache in my right shoulder and tingling in my fingers.

Conversation 2

Nurse (Woman): Mr. Johns, how bad is your chest pain now? What does it feel like?
Patient (Man): It feels like a sharp pain when I breathe in.

Conversation 3

Nurse (Woman): What's the problem with your elbow, Mr. Green?
Patient (Man): It is very painful when I straighten my arm out.
Nurse (Woman): What does the pain feel like?
Patient (Man): It feels like a stabbing pain every time I stretch my arm out.

Conversation 4

Nurse (Woman): Mr. Wilson, you told me you had a pain in your left shoulder and neck, what does the pain feel like?
Patient (Man): I don't know why, but it feels like a dull pain whenever I move my neck or arm.
Nurse (Woman): Does the pain radiate down your arm?
Patient (Man): Yes, it does sometimes.

Conversation 5

Patient (Man): I have a red rash on my body; I have had it for two days now.
Nurse (Woman): OK, Mr. Dan, is it itchy? Does it cause you any pain?
Patient (Man): No, it doesn't really hurt. It stings when I scratch it.
Nurse (Woman): Do you have any other problems?
Patient (Man): No, there is nothing else wrong.

This is the end of Part One. Now look at Part Two.
You will hear a conversation between a patient and a doctor about health problem. For each of the following sentences, decide whether it is True (A) or False (B). Put a tick (√) in the relevant box. Mark the corresponding letter on your answer sheet. You will hear the conversation twice.
Doctor (Man): Welcome, Mrs. Brown, come in and sit down here please. So, would you

please tell me your first name?

Patient (Woman): It's Casey. That's C-A-S-E-Y.

Doctor (Man): OK. What's your occupation?

Patient (Woman): Well, I'm teaching at Saint John's University and I've got pretty busy in the past month.

Doctor (Man): I understand you have a busy schedule. This Tuesday you just had a breast ultrasound and chest X-ray. Now I've got the result. From the test report, what you've got is a lump of fibrosis tissue. No real cause for worrying, but I think we should deal with it.

Patient (Woman): Oh no, is it so serious?

Doctor (Man): I'm afraid not, but it won't get better of its own accord. I would recommend you to come in and deal with the situation by operation.

Patient (Woman): Couldn't the lump be melted away by medicine?

Doctor (Man): Sorry, I don't think so. An operation is the only way to stop the problem.

Patient (Woman): Oh dear. It's not a cancer, is it?

Doctor (Man): No, it's not, but I think you'll be a lot more comfortable without the tumor there.

Patient (Woman): I suppose you know best, but to be honest, I'm extremely afraid of hospitals.

Doctor (Man): I know, Casey, but hospitals are useful places to turn to help when you need them. You'll only be in for ten days or so, and once the operation is over, you'll feel so much better. Shall I put you on the waiting list?

Patient (Woman): How long will it be?

Doctor (Man): Well, it's hard to tell now. But usually it takes about 4 months. Is that all right for your holidays?

Patient (Woman): Yes, let's get it over with before then.

Doctor (Man): Very well, Mrs. Brown. We'll wait for you to get this fixed up. Goodbye, and please don't worry too much about hospitals.

Patient (Woman): Goodbye, doctor, and thanks very much.

This is the end of Part Two. Now look at Part Three.

You will hear a conversation between a patient and a doctor about his disease. For each of the following questions or unfinished sentences, choose the correct answer A, B or C. Put a tick (√) in the relevant box. Mark the corresponding letter on your answer sheet. You will hear the conversation twice.

Doctor (Woman): Mr. Jones, I have heard that you are fond of desserts and alcohol, right?

Patient (Man): Yes, I can't go to sleep without a drink. I know that diabetic patients should not drink, but I can't resist the temptation of wine.

Doctor (Woman): Right now your blood glucose is a little bit high. If you don't give up drinking and don't stop desserts, complications will become worse. Why don't we find a way together to curb your desire for wine and desserts?
Patient (Man): That's fine. What I need is your instructions and help.
Doctor (Woman): Then let us do something interesting like listening to music, playing chess and reading novels to move your attention away from alcohol and desserts. We can plan an appropriate diet menu for you. We can also request that the nutritionist prepare food with good color and flavor for you to stimulate your appetite. I'm sure you are capable of controlling wine and desserts intake.
Patient (Man): Sure, I'll do my best to cooperate with you. Another question is that I have problems in both of my eyes. My left eye is almost totally blind and the eyesight of my right eye is also very poor. This makes it very inconvenient for me to get around. Can they be treated?
Doctor (Woman): They can be treated. We can ask the eye doctor to see you after your blood glucose level become normal. A simple operation will enable you to see again.
Patient (Man): That's great. I'll cooperate with you to have my blood glucose controlled and the schedule for the eye operation planned as soon as possible.
Doctor (Woman): Fine, let's work hard together.

This is the end of Part Three. Now look at Part Four.
You will hear a conversation between a nurse and a patient about her vital signs. Fill in the blanks. Write the answers on your answer sheet. You will hear the conversation twice.
Nurse (Man): Hi, Madam. What's your name?
Patient (Woman): I'm Jenny Thompson.
Nurse (Man): OK. Mrs. Thompson, what's your problem?
Patient (Woman): I think I might have a fever, and I coughed so much that I felt I was going to pass out. That's why I came to the emergency room.
Nurse (Man): OK. Mrs. Thompson, I'll take your vital signs first, and then you may need to do the X-ray check.
Patient (Woman): Go ahead.
Nurse (Man): I'm going to insert the probe into your mouth to measure your temperature, so raise your tongue please; it will last for three minutes to get an accurate value. During that time, please do not move your tongue or speak, OK?
Patient (Woman): All right.
Nurse (Man): Now I'm going to check your pulse for about one minute. Please give me your left hand with palm up. I'll take it by the radial site.
Patient (Woman): OK.
Nurse (Man): Now I want to take your blood pressure. Please follow my directions and

just relax. OK. Mrs. Thompson, since you are a little short of breath, I also need to take your oxygen saturation. Please give me your left index finger. I'll put a clamp on it, but don't be nervous, it won't hurt. The infrared sensor in the clamp will get the blood oxygen saturation in your capillary.

Patient (Woman): OK. Thank you.

Nurse (Man): Mrs. Thompson, your temperature is 39 ℃; pulse is 110 bpm, regular; respiration is 35 bpm, regular but shallow and quick; BP is 120/80 mmHg; oxygen saturation is 90%. It seems that you need a further examination. Dr. Steven will follow up your case. Please be seated and do not stop the oxygen.

Patient (Woman): OK. Thank you very much.

This is the end of Part Four. You now have five minutes to write your answers on the answer sheet. You have one more minute. This is the end of the listening test.

参考答案及解析

Ⅰ Listening

Part One

1. E 病人右肩感觉疼痛(aching),手指有刺痛感(tingling),故选 E。

2. H 病人自述呼吸时能感觉胸口的尖锐痛(sharp pain),故选 H。

3. D 病人每次伸展胳膊时都能感觉尖锐的刺痛(stabbing pain),故选 D。

4. A 病人自述每当移动脖子或手臂时感觉到钝痛(dull pain),故选 A。

5. B 病人身体有皮疹,每次抓挠时有刺痛(sting),故选 B。

Part Two

6. B 病人患有纤维化组织硬块(lump of fibrosis tissue),但并不严重,故本句错误。

7. A 硬块不会自行消失,也无法通过药物清除,唯一的方法是手术治疗,故本句正确。

8. A 医生告诉病人这只是肿瘤(tumor),不是癌症,故本句正确。

9. B 病人说她害怕住院(afraid of hospitals),并未感觉轻松(at ease),故本句错误。

10. A 病人同意将其名字加入手术等待名单(waiting list),故本句正确。

Part Three

11. B 病人自述是糖尿病患者(diabetic patient),故选 B。

12. B 医生告知病人如果不戒酒(drinking wine)、不停止进甜食(dessert),并发症会加重,故选 B。

13. C 医生建议通过听音乐、下象棋、读小说的方式转移注意力,故选 C。

14. A 病人自述还有另外一个病情,即视力(eyesight)很不好,故选 A。

15. C 医生说通过眼部手术可以改善病人视力欠佳的问题,但在手术之前需要将病人的血糖控制好,将其恢复至正常水平,故选 C。

Part Four

16. coughed　在对话开头部分,病人说她可能发烧,咳嗽得很厉害,以至于差点晕倒。

17. temperature　护士告诉病人会将口温探测器(probe)放进其口腔测量体温。

18. pulse　护士要求病人伸出左手,掌心朝上,测量她的桡动脉处脉搏。

19. oxygen　护士发现病人呼吸短促(short of breath),决定测量她的氧饱和度(oxygen saturation)。

20. regular　测量结果显示病人的呼吸频率比较规律(regular),但是呼吸较浅且急促(shallow and quick)。

Ⅱ　Reading and Writing

Part One

21. C　可以利用humidifier快速找到原文C段中的文字,即"A humidifier puts more moisture in the air."

22. A　根据reading or watching TV很容易就能找到原文A段信息"If you notice your eyes are dry mainly while reading or watching TV ..."得出由看电视导致的眼部干燥。

23. B　根据excessive air movement可以找到原文B段的文字"Excessive air movement dries out your eyes."

24. D　由warm compresses和inflammation of the eyelids分别可以定位原文D段第一和第二句话,即"Warm compresses and eyelid scrubs with baby shampoo help provide ... This is especially helpful if you have inflammation of the eyelids or problems ..."第一句说热敷以及使用婴儿香波对眼睑进行冲洗,有助于眼部润滑层的生成,而第二句进一步提到这种方法对于眼睑的炎症特别有效。

25. F　根据lubricating eye ointments and eyedrops可以找到原文F段,即"Lubricating eye ointments are much thicker than eyedrops and gels."该句提到了具有润滑作用的眼膏比滴眼液粘稠得多,然后在第二句中又进一步说明了眼膏因为粘稠,所以比滴眼液持续的时间要久。这些都是对眼膏和滴眼液的差别在进行比较。

26. E　由artificial tears and lubricating eyedrops可以定位原文E段,即"Artificial tears and lubricating eyedrops and gels (available over the counter) help ...",说明了人造泪液和润滑性滴眼液的用途。

27. D　根据glands和massaging可以找到原文D段,即"the massaging action helps draw the oil out of the glands"说明按摩有助于将油从腺体中排除。

28. B　根据ceiling fans可以找到原文B段,即"Avoid this by decreasing the speed of ceiling fans and/or oscillating fans."说明了降低吊扇的风速可以避免眼部干燥。

29. C　根据air conditioners可以找到原文中C段的"Also, both furnaces and air conditioners decrease humidity in the air"说明空调能降低空气中的湿度。

30. F　根据eye oinments可以定位原文F段,该段第三句和第四句,即"However, because of their thickness, ointments may blur your vision if used during the day. Therefore, they are typically used to lubricate the eyes overnight while you sleep."说明白天使用眼膏可能会影响视线,因此通常在晚上睡觉的时候使用,对应了题干中所指的使用

眼膏的恰当时间。

Part Two

31. A　题干的重点是“do not seek medical advice”，这与文章第一段第一句，即“do not consult a doctor”意思相同，故本题正确。

32. B　题干的意思是由于误诊，50％的偏头痛患者未能获得对症的治疗，而文章第一段第二句中指出“... 50％ of migraine sufferers had not sought medical advice and had not been diagnosed with migraine. As a result, they were not being treated for migraine.”即50％的偏头痛患者没有去问诊，未被诊断为偏头痛才导致了没有对症治疗，故本题错。

33. B　题干的意思是亲友们的同情能够缓解疼痛，而文章第二段的第二句“They may receive sympathy from relatives, friends and colleagues but this does not ease the pain.”正好与题干意思相反，故本题错。

34. A　题干的意思是发生剧烈的头痛并伴有眩晕的时候，应该及时向医生报告，文中第三段的第二句话，即“Any severe or constant headache that begins suddenly and is accompanied by weakness, dizziness, numbness or other strange physical sensations should be reported to a doctor immediately.”表达的是相同的含义，故本题正确。

35. C　题干的意思是在停止使用止痛药物之前应该向医生咨询，而文章第四段第一句中仅提到了“Your doctor should be consulted if you have frequent debilitating headaches or take an excessive number of pain relievers.”即过度服用止疼药物的情况下，应该向医生咨询，并未提到题干中的内容，故选C。

36. A　题干的意思是医生会就如何合理用药给你建议，虽然文中没有直接出现题干中的内容，但是从第五段的前两句，即“The role of your doctor is to accurately diagnose your headache and then to work with you to help minimize the effect it has on you and your lifestyle. Recommending medication is a part of this process.”可以看出，医生的职责是正确地诊断头痛，然后和你一起将头痛对你和你的生活所产生的影响降到最低，而药物的推荐则是这个过程中的一部分，故本题正确。

37. A　题干的意思是你应该告诉你的医生头痛是如何影响到你的生活和你的朋友的，第五段的最后一句“Make sure your doctor is aware of the disability caused by headache to your quality of life and how it affects your partner, children, employer, work colleagues and friends.”即应该确保你的医生了解头痛对你的生活质量所造成的影响，以及头痛是如何影响到你的伴侣、孩子、老板、同事和朋友的，故本题正确。

38. B　题干意思是控制头痛并非难事，因为你有多种治疗的方案可供选择，但文章第六段的第一句便指出“Headache management is a great challenge.”说明了控制头痛是相当大的挑战，虽然在第二句中提到了“A number of treatment options ...”，但是在后续的内容中却说“... may have to be tried to discover what works best for each headache sufferer.”即要找到最适合你的治疗方案，需要经过许多次的尝试，所以本题错。

39. A　题干意思是医生在分辨哪种方案对治疗你的头痛最有效的过程中十分重要，第六段的第二句和第三句中提到“A number of treatment options, preparations and methods of administration may have to be tried to discover what works best for each headache sufferer. The role of the doctor is vital in this process.”即头痛患者可能不得不

尝试各种各样的治疗选择、准备和管理办法,从而找出最适合自己的那种,而医生在这个过程中起到重要的作用,故本题正确。

40. A　题干的意思是有效的医患沟通将能获取有效的治疗效果,最后一段的第一句和第二句便提到了"Patient-doctor communication is vital for the best outcome. Effective communication on both sides can result in ... that will minimize the pain and disability associated with headache."即医患交流对于最佳的治疗效果来说的重要性,故本题正确。

Part Three

41. B　文章第一段的最后一句中提到"It seems that about one in ten of people over 65 feel chronically lonely all or most of the time."即 65 岁以上的人,大约十个人中就有一个人大部分时间或始终感受到长期的孤独。十个中有一个即为百分之十的比例,故选 B。

42. B　文章的第二段分析了导致老年人孤独的两个原因,即"easy transport ... and the ability to make arrangements online ..."分别指便利的交通和使用网络来安排生活的能力,故选 B。

43. A　文章第三段的第二句话中指出"A lack of social connections is 'a risk factor for early death', which can be compared to smoking 15 cigarettes a day ..."即缺少社交联络是导致提前死亡的危险因素之一,相当于每天吸 15 支烟,题干中的"heavy smoking"就相当于文中的"smoking 15 cigarettes a day",故选 A。

44. C　该题题干问,第四段中的 stigma 一词是什么意思。stigma 一词本意为耻辱或污名。但是如果不知道该词什么意思的话,可以根据上下文来进行推测。在文章第四段第一句中 stigma 和 negative attitude 是用 and 来连接的,由此可以推断出它们之间在含义上是并列关系,stigma 应该是一个贬义的词。选项 A 表示有利的,选项 B 表示值得骄傲的,选项 C 表示丢人的,通过排除法,便可以得出,应该选 C。

45. B　选项 A 出现在第一段的第二句中"... but here and now old people are more likely to be bitterly lonely, according to a paper by Marcus Rand of *The Campaign to End Loneliness*",这是 Marcus Rand 提出的。选项 C 出现在最后一段"The irony of all this is that those who may be old and lonely now are the ones who may well have thought in 1960s that youth and only youth was worth living or thinking about."这是现在这些孤独的老人在二十世纪六十年代的时候,也就是他们年轻的时候所持的观点。选项 B 出现在第四段"... there's nothing wrong with admitting to being lonely, and things can be done to help reduce it ...",这是直接引用 Morrison 的话,表示应该采取措施来缓解孤独感,故选 B。

Part Four

46. B　由第一步"准备使用除颤器"和第三步"打开除颤器"得知,第二步应该是使用前的注意事项,选项 B 表达的正是"在使用除颤器前,应将病人移到干燥的地方,避免除颤时遇水导电"。

47. F　这一步骤指导如何将除颤仪电极片正确贴到病人身上,将其中一片贴片贴在病人右胸乳头上方位置,接下去应该是选项 F"将另一片贴片轻轻贴在左胸腔乳头下方位置"。找到上一句中的"one pad"和选项 F 中的"the other pad"是解题的关键。

48. C　由后文"在机器检测病人心律时不要触碰病人"得知,检测心律是自动除颤仪在分析病人是否要接受除颤,所以正确答案应该是选项 C"按下自动除颤仪的分析按钮进行检测,并且不要触碰病人”。

49. E 前一步是“按下除颤按钮”,在对病人进行除颤后,应立即为其实施 5 个循环大约 2 分钟的心脏按压,选项 E 中的 shock 与前一步骤的 shock 正好是上下承接的关系,故选 E。

50. A 最后一步表达的是术后应注意的事项,选项 A 提醒,即使病人已经苏醒,“在医疗救援人员到达前,不要拆下电极片或断开除颤仪和电极片的连接”。

Part Five

51. D 由上文“... is difficulty in remembering recent events”可以得知记忆有困难,是一种记忆力的丧失,故选 loss(丧失)。

52. B 此处表达“……的丧失”应为名词,由上文得知此处表示阿尔茨海默症的各类症状,其中包括“丧失动力”,故选 motivation(动力)。

53. K 此处表达“……的速度”应为名词,由上文得知“身体的技能逐渐丧失最终死亡”,这是一段发展过程,故选 progression(发展,进程)。

54. F 由后文“genes”得知阿尔茨海默症有部分原因是由基因引起的,所以此处应该选跟基因相关的词 genetic(基因的)。

55. C 此处表达的内容是关于阿尔茨海默症的诊断,是基于病史和认知测试等情况的,be based on 是固定词组搭配,意为“以……为根据”,故选 C。

56. J 这句话中的 mistake 说明阿尔茨海默症最初容易被误诊,而其主要症状就是记忆力衰退、无法自理等,这跟衰老后出现的症状是相似的,故选 ageing(老化,变老)。

57. I 此处应该填写一个动词搭配后面的名词 risk(风险),由上文得知,多动脑子、多运动、防止肥胖都是属于能减少得病风险的,故选 decrease(减少)。

58. A 此处 or 表示这个单词和 stop 是并列关系而且意思相近,因为句子的意思是表示“没有治疗方法能停止或逆转病情的发展”,故以选 reverse(倒转)。

59. G 此处单词修饰的是 elements(因素),所以应该是个形容词,上文讲到压力包括的几个因素有社会上的、精神上的、身体上,故选 economic(经济上的)。

60. E 由后文 improve(改善)得知这个锻炼方法应该是有利的,故选 beneficial(有利的)。

Part Six

61.

Discharge Summary

Martin Downes, a 43-year-old male patient, was hospitalized on April 24th, 2017 with a complaint of repeated cough and fever for 20 days. He also complained that he had urinary frequency and urgency for 4 days. Examination on admission showed that there was harsh respiratory sound in his lungs and heart murmurs. He was diagnosed with interstitial pneumonia and urinary tract infection, accompanied by secondary fungus infection.

On this diagnosis, he received anti-infection and anti-virus treatment in order to eliminate phlegm, improve immunity and alleviate fungus infection. The result of the treatment was very good and the patient was discharged on May 1st, 2017 in stable conditions.

No medications are needed after discharge, but the patient needs to drink enough water and take enough rest to prevent the recurrence of the disease.

【审题】

这是一篇关于出院小结的作文。要求考生写 100 词左右的出院记录,将表格中的信息整理成文字进行描述,内容应包括:病人姓名、年龄、性别、入院时间、出院时间、症状、诊断、治疗、医嘱等。表格中的信息要尽量表述完整,无遗漏;语言表达尽量简明扼要,并注意适当运用一些常见的表达用语,如:be admitted to the hospital /be hospitalized; with a complaint of /complain that; be diagnosed with; accompanied by 等。

【范文评述】

本篇范文内容详实,涵盖了试题中提供的所有细节,包括病人的基本信息、入院出院时间、症状、诊断、治疗方法及医嘱等。语言通顺,无病句或其他语法错误。时态使用正确,如第一、二段主要用过去时,因陈述过去的事实,如第一段提到的入院时间、主诉、诊断等;第二段提到病人所接受的治疗、效果等;而第三段则主要使用一般现在时,因其内容为病人出院后的医嘱。在语言使用上也有亮点如:第一段提到病人主诉时,为避免重复,用到了"with a complaint of ..."和"complain that ..."两种句型;有效应用一些词组来连接上下文,如"accompanied by ...""On this diagnosis""in order to"及"in case of"等,使行文更紧凑。